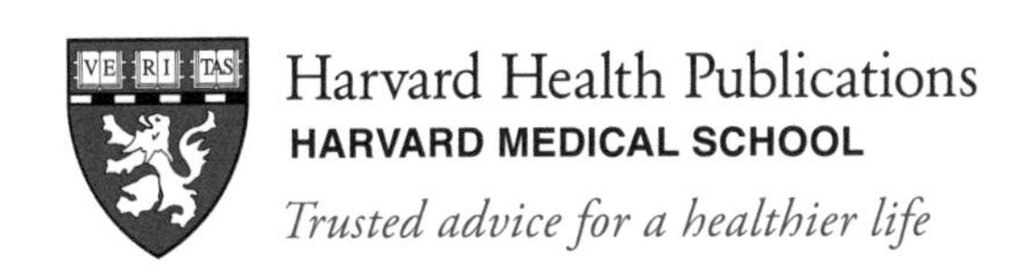

Dear Reader,

Does your neck feel stiff when you awaken in the morning? Or do the muscles seize painfully with no warning? Maybe a dull ache and tightness in your neck and upper back is a constant companion?

If you're bothered by neck pain, you have plenty of company. In a recent three-month period, about 15% of adults in the United States experienced neck pain, according to the Centers for Disease Control and Prevention. Doctors estimate that seven out of 10 people will be troubled by it at some point in their lives. For one in 20, it is longstanding and intense enough to severely limit the ability to work and play. Unfortunately, neck pain usually recurs. Between 50% and 85% of people who experience it will be bothered by it again within the next five years.

Why is pain in the neck area so common? Your neck must be strong enough to support a heavy weight—your head—but must still allow you to tilt, turn, and nod your head easily. This combination of strength and flexibility requires a complex system of muscles, bones, tendons, and nerves. As a result, the neck is vulnerable to strain and injury.

The good news is that neck pain, although painful and limiting, is rarely a serious medical problem. Except in unusual cases, it is not dangerous and does not lead to disability. And while medicine cannot yet offer a cure for many types of chronic neck pain, other types are often short-lived. No matter which type you suffer from, there are many things you and your doctor can do to manage and relieve the pain, including a combination of self-help techniques and over-the-counter pain medications.

One important shift in the field is that people with neck pain now play an increasingly active role in their own recovery. For example, treatments that used to be common, such as lengthy bed rest or wearing a neck collar, have been replaced by encouragement to return to a normal routine as soon as possible with the help of physical therapy and medications. A program that emphasizes stretching, strengthening, and staying active can help relieve neck pain and prevent it from recurring in the future. Less commonly, surgery is needed to provide relief.

This report will cover the most common causes of neck pain. You will learn about diagnostic methods, treatment options, and simple steps you can take to ease and manage the aches—and deal effectively with that pain in your neck.

Sincerely,

Robert H. Shmerling, M.D.
Medical Editor

Where bone, muscle, and nerve converge

The neck is a remarkable and underappreciated part of the body. Every segment of the scaffolding that supports it—vertebrae, muscles, ligaments, and joints—works with the others in carefully coordinated ways to function so smoothly that most of the time, you're not even aware of your neck—that is, until something goes wrong.

Most neck pain begins in the uppermost part of the spine, known as the cervical spine, and its supporting structures. This area is so vulnerable because of the nature of the tasks it has to perform and their requirements for both strength and precision. The neck supports the roughly 11 pounds of your head. Imagine how tired your arm would be if you had to hold even a light umbrella up for 18 hours a day. Your neck supports a much heavier weight all day, every day, whether you're staring straight ahead at the computer screen, gazing up at the stars, or looking down at a book.

Figure 1: Where it hurts—bones and nerves

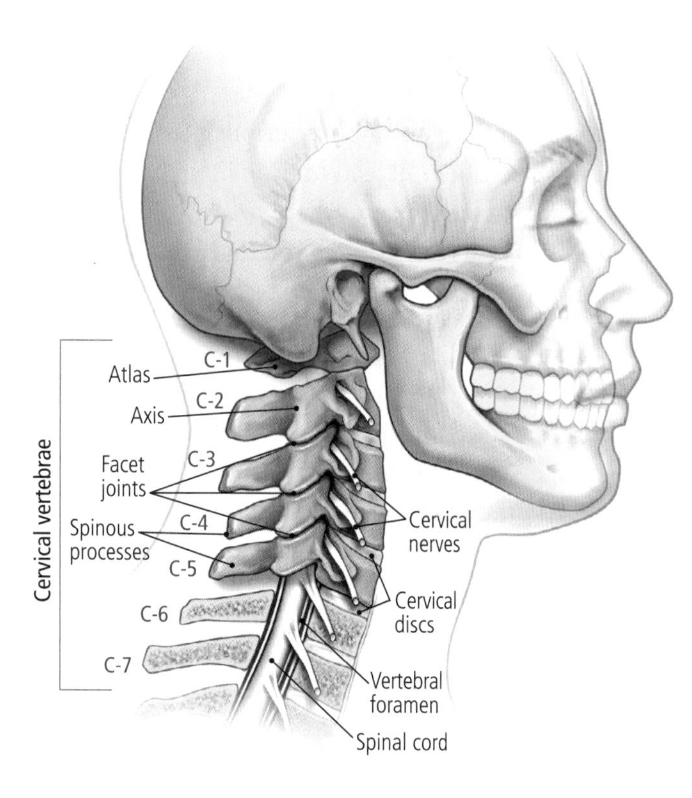

Your neck's intricate scaffolding of bones and nerves provides support for your head and protection for your spinal column. But an area with so many interacting parts is ripe for problems. Bones may compress delicate nerves, joints can deteriorate, and discs can bulge, causing discomfort and pain.

At the same time, it must be able to rotate your head from left to right in addition to positioning it up or down—and it has to handle all these movements as smoothly as the Steadicam on a movie set.

Finally, the cervical spine must protect your spinal cord, which contains the vital nerves that carry messages from your brain to the rest of your body. Unlike your skull, which easily protects your brain because it is rigid, your neck must shield the spinal cord while permitting a great deal of movement.

Unfortunately, the intricate anatomy required to fulfill these tasks makes the neck prone to injury. This chapter explores that anatomy and briefly explains why each of the structures in the neck can cause pain.

The bones

The great mobility of your neck is accomplished by seven interlocking bones called the cervical vertebrae, which constitute your cervical spine (see Figure 1, at left). The first cervical vertebra, known as C-1, sits at the top of the spine, supporting the bottom of your skull. The seventh, the C-7 vertebra, can be felt as the prominent bump at the bottom of your neck.

Each vertebra consists of two parts—a rounded bony part in the front (shaped like a hockey puck) and an arch of bone in the back surrounding a hole, called the vertebral foramen (plural: foramina). If you can imagine the seven vertebrae stacked one on top of the other, you will see that the holes line up to form the vertebral canal. The spinal cord passes through this canal. In addition, the vertebrae are shaped so that there are narrow openings on the sides where each vertebra meets its upper and lower neighbors. Through these gaps, eight pairs of spinal nerves exit the spinal column and extend to areas of your upper body.

Despite these similarities, the seven vertebrae in the cervical spine are not identical.

- The C-1 vertebra—a ring-shaped bone that supports and balances the skull—is aptly named the atlas, after the Greek god who shouldered the weight of the world. Curves on the bottom of the back section of your skull fit into shallow grooves in the C-1 vertebra, forming the flexible joint that lets you nod your head "yes."
- Below it, the C-2 vertebra, called the axis, has an extension that sticks up through an opening in the atlas; called the dens, or odontoid process, this extension provides the base around which your neck pivots as you shake your head "no."
- C-7 is also distinct. It's known as the vertebra prominens because of the long bony extension (or spinous process) at the back of the bone. Most people can feel this through their skin.
- The remaining vertebrae—C-3 through C-6—are not known by other names and are structured more like vertebrae lower in the spine. Each allows a relatively small amount of movement, but together they enable you to rotate or bend your head to the side and move it forward and backward.

How the bones can cause problems: The vertebrae provide excellent protection for the nerves, but space is tight, and the nerves sometimes become pinched between the bones, causing pain in the neck or difficulty in movement or sensation in the regions served by the nerves.

Connectors: Discs and facet joints

What's to keep the vertebrae from scraping against one another while you nod your head and twist your neck? Between each pair of vertebrae is an intervertebral disc, along with two facet joints that connect and protect the bones while permitting some degree of movement.

Intervertebral discs

Most people have heard of intervertebral discs (if only in the context of a "herniated disc" or "ruptured disc"). These cushioning discs, which consist primarily of cartilage, separate the bodies of the vertebrae, absorb shock, and prevent the bones from scraping against one another.

A normal disc has a gel-like center and a tougher outer covering, called the annulus, that binds the vertebrae together. The squishy interior lets the disc change shape in response to pressure. This allows the vertebrae to move relative to one another as you flex and extend your neck.

How the discs can cause problems: With age, discs become thinner, stiffer, and drier. This reduces their ability to absorb shocks and makes them more vulnerable to damage, such as rupturing or bulging.

Facet joints

The bony arch at the back of each vertebra is connected to the neighboring vertebra's arch by a pair of small joints called facet joints. Something like the connections between train cars, facet joints hook the vertebrae together but allow a controlled degree of movement in between. Cumulatively, the small movements permitted by each cervical facet joint allow you to bend your neck forward, backward, and to the side. The facet joints are about the size of your little finger's knuckles and are contained within protective joint capsules filled with lubricating fluid called synovial fluid.

How the facet joints can cause problems: Facet joints are rich in nerve endings, which signal pain if the joint is squeezed or jerked past its normal range of motion, as might occur in an auto accident. The joints can also become sore when held at the extreme of their normal range for long periods, as might happen when you spend an afternoon painting the ceiling.

Like joints elsewhere in the body, the facet joints are subject to damage from rheumatoid arthritis (the inflammation of joints) or osteoarthritis (the gradual breakdown or "wear and tear" of cartilage in the joints), either of which can be the source of neck pain (see "Cervical osteoarthritis," page 13).

Muscles, tendons, and ligaments

The stack of vertebrae and discs in your neck would quickly topple without muscles and other tissues holding them in place. But these, too, can cause trouble.

Muscles

About two dozen large and small muscles in the neck, upper back, and shoulders help support the cervical spine and keep it aligned properly, while allowing a great deal of movement. Some muscles have a single function, but most help you move in several directions.

In the back of your neck are a group of posterior, or extensor, muscles that contract when you extend your neck. Of these extensor muscles, your trapezius muscles are the largest and most noticeable. They run down the back of your neck and fan out toward your shoulders (see Figure 2, below).

Toward the front, your anterior, or flexor, muscles help balance and stabilize your head. You can feel them work if you lie on your back and slightly lift your head off the floor (without tilting it forward). Compared with the posterior neck muscles, the anterior muscles are relatively small and weak—particularly in people with neck pain.

Lateral muscles help balance your head and let you bend it to the side. And the muscles of your shoulders and upper back, particularly those between your shoulder blades, form an important base that supports the neck and head.

How the muscles can cause problems: If you commonly stand, drive, or do desk work with your head out in front, rather than directly balanced over your spine, your posterior neck muscles must stay contracted in order to keep your head upright. And that can spell trouble. Although the muscles are quite strong, they may not withstand such prolonged effort for very long before they begin to ache. Both the anterior and lateral muscles are easily overstretched and injured in a whiplash-type accident, and they readily tighten to cause neck pain.

In fact, injury or overuse of any of the neck muscles can cause pain. Even sleeping in an awkward position or simply sitting at a desk all day can lead to muscle strain and pain. And this can set up ripple effects. Muscle weakness in one or more muscle groups can make it difficult to maintain a healthy posture, which in turn puts added stress on the discs and joints of the spine.

Figure 2: Where it hurts—muscles of the neck

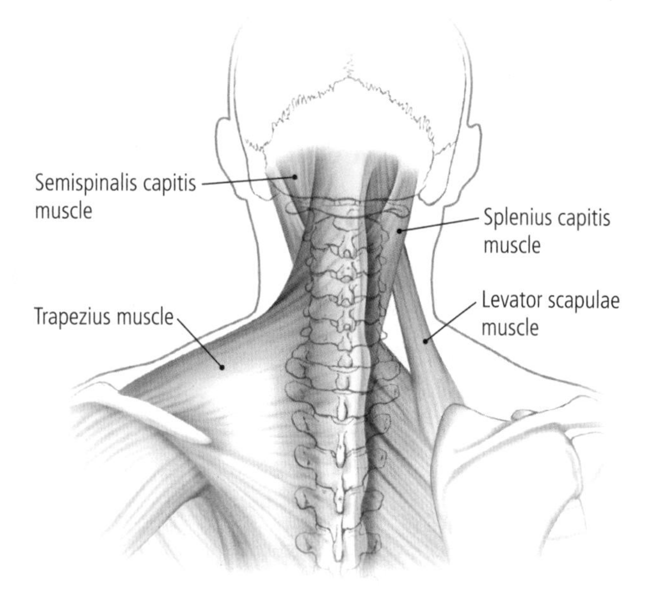

The posterior (rear) neck muscles do the lion's share of work in supporting the weight of your head while it tilts and turns. Pain can occur when injury strains or tears neck muscles, but more often, aches and pains result when muscles tense and strain to protect neck joints and nerves that have deteriorated. The brawny trapezius muscle is one of the most common sites of neck pain and strain.

Tendons and ligaments

What holds it all together? Tendons are the strong, flexible cords that make up the attachments between neck muscles and bones—the cervical spine, collarbones, ribs, shoulder blades, and head. The whole system of bones, joints, and muscles is reinforced and stabilized by more rigid bands of tissue called ligaments, which connect bones to one another and help prevent excessive movement that can cause damage. Short ligaments connect adjoining cervical vertebrae, while longer ligaments extend along the entire cervical spine.

How tendons and ligaments can cause problems: Tendons are really just extensions of muscle and are vulnerable to the same types of strains as the muscles to which they're attached. Acute neck pain, for example, can be caused by tendinitis (inflammation of a tendon) rather than damage to the main part of the muscle. In addition, ligaments can be sprained by overstretching or microscopic tears.

Other structures

The neck is complicated and crowded with structures unrelated to the musculoskeletal system. Neck pain is sometimes a symptom of problems with the arteries supplying blood to the brain (which go through holes in the vertebrae), the thyroid gland, the trachea (windpipe), the lymph nodes, or the esophagus.

Shoulder connections: How the neck and shoulders interact

The neck and shoulders are separate entities, with, for the most part, separate muscles, joints, and ligaments controlling their respective movements. However, they are close collaborators, and it can sometimes be tough to know where neck pain ends and shoulder pain begins.

The trapezius muscles

If you feel an ache in both your neck and shoulders, there's a good chance that the source of the pain is the trapezius muscles (see Figure 2, page 4). The trapezius muscles are true multitaskers. They work with upper back and neck muscles to support your head and neck while collaborating with more than a dozen shoulder muscles to stabilize and move the large triangular shoulder blades. Each shoulder blade (scapula) provides a connection between your upper arm bone (humerus) and collarbone (clavicle).

The trapezius muscles are among 30 different muscles that work with key ligaments and tendons to provide movement and support for the entire shoulder. The majority of those muscles enable the shoulder joint—the most mobile joint in the body—to move in a variety of ways. Four rotator cuff muscles surrounding the joint enable you to raise your arm from your side and rotate your shoulder in many directions. The large, robust deltoid muscle enables you to lift your arm, once it's away from your side, and the pectoralis major stabilizes the arm and allows you to move the arm across the chest.

How the trapezius muscles can cause problems: These muscles are not directly involved with moving your head and neck, but there is a delicate balance between the neck and shoulder muscles, and a shoulder problem can upset that balance and strain a muscle in your neck.

The brachial plexus

The neck and shoulders are also connected through a network of nerves called the brachial plexus. The roots of these nerves are located at the cervical spine. They exit through the spaces between the cervical vertebrae and join together to provide sensation to the shoulder and the entire arm. Each nerve root is named for the cervical vertebra at which it exits. For example, the C-4 nerve root exits above the C-4 vertebra.

How the brachial plexus can cause problems: Injuries to the brachial plexus are common in contact sports, particularly football and wrestling, and cause a burning or stinging sensation radiating from the shoulders down the arm. They can also produce neck pain if the injury occurs closer to where the nerve exits the spinal column. ■

Evaluating neck pain

It's essential to see a doctor about your neck pain so that you can get an accurate diagnosis. However, diagnosing neck problems can be challenging. Even after a rigorous medical workup, you may receive no specific explanation for your pain, and your treatment may be aimed at relieving the discomfort and helping you function normally rather than repairing an underlying anatomical problem.

Neck pain is treated by a number of medical specialists (see "What type of doctor should I see for my neck pain?" on page 7). But be aware that specialists generally look first for the conditions they understand best. For example, a neurologist may be more likely to test for nerve pain. So, it is usually a good idea to start with your primary care doctor, who can set you in the right direction and help determine which specialist, if any, you might need.

When to seek immediate medical attention

Most neck pain doesn't stem from anything medically serious, making it safe to try self-care strategies before seeking medical help. However, if your neck pain is so severe you can't sit still, or if it is accompanied by any of the following symptoms, contact a medical professional right away:

- ✔ **Fever, headache, and neck stiffness.** This triad of symptoms might indicate bacterial meningitis, an infection of the spinal cord and brain covering that requires prompt treatment with antibiotics.
- ✔ **Pain traveling down one arm,** especially if the arm or hand is weak, numb, or tingling. Your symptoms might indicate that a herniated cervical disc is pressing on a nerve.
- ✔ **Loss of bowel or bladder control.** This might indicate pressure on the spinal cord or spinal nerve roots, needing immediate attention.
- ✔ **Extreme instability.** If you can suddenly flex or extend your neck much farther than usual, it might indicate a fracture or torn ligaments. This usually occurs only after significant impact or injury, and is more likely to be detected by your doctor or on an x-ray than by your own perception.
- ✔ **Persistent swollen glands in the neck.** Infection or tumor can result in swollen glands and neck pain.
- ✔ **Chest pain or pressure.** A heart attack or inflamed heart muscle can cause neck pain along with more classic heart symptoms.

Describing your pain

When you see the doctor, it's best to be as clear as you can in describing what your pain feels like. With so many things that can go wrong, there are clearly many possibilities to consider—and people may perceive the same type of pain differently. Before your appointment, think about how you would describe your neck pain. Are your neck and shoulders stiff? Do you feel a sharp pain or hear a grinding noise when you turn your head? Pain can be mild or severe, achy or sharp, stationary or shooting. It may stand alone or be accompanied by other troublesome complaints. By clearly describing your specific neck symptom—or combination of symptoms, because they often overlap—you can help your doctor determine what's wrong and how to help.

Types of pain

The following descriptions of different types of pain will help you clearly explain your symptoms.

Muscle pain. Aching or sore neck and shoulder muscles may occur in response to overexertion, prolonged physical stress (usually from poor neck positioning during everyday activities), or emotional tension. Muscles may also develop hard knots that are sore to the touch.

Muscle spasm. This is a sudden, powerful contraction of neck muscles. When you wake up with a painful stiff neck, that's likely a muscle spasm—what is sometimes called a "crick" in your neck. The muscle usually feels painful, tight, or knotted, and may be impossible to move. Muscle spasm can result from a

What type of doctor should I see for my neck pain?

Many types of health professionals are trained to help manage neck pain. Which specialist you see depends largely on the underlying cause of your pain.

Often the best place to start is with your primary care doctor, who can evaluate your condition, order a variety of tests, and prescribe treatment. Frequently, your doctor will refer you to a physical therapist (see "Choosing a physical therapist," page 20). If your doctor decides you need more advanced, targeted care, he or she will refer you to any one of the following specialists:

Neurologist. A neurologist specializes in diagnosing and treating disorders of the nervous system, including diseases of the brain, spinal cord, nerves, and muscles. A neurologist may be involved in your care if your neck pain is caused by any number of spine problems that involve the spinal nerves. Neurologists may serve as consultants to other physicians as well as providing long-term care to people with chronic neurological conditions.

Orthopedic surgeon (orthopedist). This type of doctor specializes in diagnosing and treating injuries and diseases of the musculoskeletal system with medication, exercise, surgery, or other therapeutic methods. Orthopedists tend to further specialize in certain areas of the body. For neck pain, you may be referred to an orthopedist who specializes in spinal injuries and conditions.

Osteopathic physician (osteopath). A doctor of osteopathic medicine (D.O.) diagnoses and treats conditions affecting muscles, ligaments, nerves, and joints. Osteopaths are trained to treat the body as a whole, but some have a specialization such as surgery, much like a medical doctor (M.D.). Treatment provided by an osteopath typically involves a hands-on technique known as osteopathic manipulative treatment (also called OMT or manipulation), to correct imbalances in the various musculoskeletal structures.

Physiatrist. A physiatrist is a medical doctor who has completed training in the specialty of physical medicine and rehabilitation. Physiatrists are sometimes known as rehabilitation physicians. They develop treatment plans aimed at reducing pain and restoring function lost through injury, illness, or a disabling condition.

Rheumatologist. Rheumatic diseases are painful conditions that affect joints, muscles, and bones and sometimes internal organs such as the kidneys, lungs, blood vessels, and brain. A rheumatologist specializes in diagnosing and treating these complex diseases, many of which affect structures of the neck, including rheumatoid arthritis, osteoarthritis, fibromyalgia and other pain syndromes, and musculoskeletal pain disorders.

Spine surgeon. If you are a candidate for surgery, you will be referred to a spine surgeon. Spine surgeons are typically orthopedists, neurosurgeons, or osteopathic physicians who complete additional training in spine surgery beyond their surgical residencies.

muscle injury, but it may also occur if there is a deeper problem (say, in a disc or nerve) and the muscle tenses in order to stabilize the neck and prevent you from moving in a way to cause pain or further damage. Neck muscle spasms sometimes accompany emotional stress, but often there is no identifiable reason for muscle spasm.

Headache. Neck-related headache (technically known as cervicogenic or cervical headache), is most often felt in the back of the head and upper neck, where muscles extending along the skull lie alongside neck muscles that may become tense or go into spasm. The pain is typically dull or aching, rather than sharp. It is aggravated by neck movement and often accompanied by stiffness and tenderness of neck muscles.

Facet joint pain. Often described as deep, sharp, or aching, facet joint pain typically worsens if you lean your head toward the affected side, and may radiate to your shoulder or upper back. Arthritis in the facet joints, as in other locations, may feel worse in the morning or after a period of inactivity.

Nerve pain. Irritation or pinching of the roots of the spinal nerves causes pain that may be sharp, fleeting, severe, or accompanied by pins and needles. Depending on the nerve involved, the pain may shoot down the arm or even into the hand.

Referred pain. Sometimes you feel pain at a site other than where the actual problem lies; this pain is said to be "referred." You may feel pain in your neck from shoulder damage; conversely, what you feel as pain in your shoulder, head, arms, hands, or chest may actually be referred pain from your neck. A variety of conditions can cause referred neck pain. For example, neck pain that worsens with exertion may indicate a heart problem, while pain when you eat may stem from a problem in the esophagus.

Bone pain. Pain and tenderness in the cervical vertebrae are far less common than neck pain from

Classifying neck pain

The Neck Pain Task Force, representing a number of specialties and institutions, recommends a classification system for neck pain based on medical history and physical exam. It is intended to help physicians determine the urgency of care and the appropriate diagnostic and treatment options. These are the neck pain classifications:

▾ Grade 1
No signs of a major underlying problem (such as fracture) and little interference with daily activities.

Recommendation:
No further imaging or laboratory tests are needed. The person should remain as active as possible.

▾ Grade 2
No signs of a major underlying problem, but neck pain does interfere with daily activities.

Recommendation:
In the early stages, additional imaging or laboratory tests are not necessary; treatment should focus on short-term management of symptoms.

▾ Grade 3
Neck pain with neurological signs or symptoms, such as cervical radiculopathy (see page 15).

Recommendation:
Focus should be on short-term management of symptoms; close monitoring; and CT, MRI, or electrodiagnostic tests in people with severe or progressive symptoms.

▾ Grade 4
Neck pain with a major underlying problem such as fracture, myelopathy, tumor, or infection.

Recommendation:
Test as needed to quickly determine the underlying problem and treat it appropriately.

the soft tissues. Bone pain needs medical evaluation because it can stem from serious conditions such as cancer or an infection.

Non-pain symptoms

The following symptoms may accompany neck pain or may stand alone.

Stiffness. A feeling of tightness and rigidity in the muscles can occur for a variety of reasons. It can be caused by something as simple as sleeping in an awkward position or with an unfamiliar pillow—or it can be a symptom of a serious neck injury, arthritis, or meningitis (inflammation of the lining of the brain and spinal cord). Whatever the cause, bending or moving the neck may be difficult or result in sharp pain.

Limited range of motion. With age, your ability to flex and extend your neck and bend or rotate your head from side to side may diminish somewhat, but an extremely limited or recently reduced range of motion calls for investigation (see "How far should it go?" on page 9). A limited range of motion may be short-lived, such as that caused by muscle spasm that follows an injury, or more long-lasting, such as that from joint, bone, or nerve problems.

Dizziness. When dizziness stems from a neck problem, it is called cervical vertigo. The world may spin when you move your neck, or you may feel unsteady or lightheaded. The joints of your cervical vertebrae contain position detectors that send signals to your brain to help maintain balance and coordinate your movements. If these detectors are disturbed by injury, you may feel dizzy or clumsy, in addition to feeling neck pain.

Your medical history

During the exam, your doctor will seek details about your current pain, other neck symptoms, and many aspects of your life and medical history. Be prepared to answer questions such as these:

- Did the pain come on suddenly or over time? Is it constant or does it come and go?
- Did anything happen that may have brought it on? For instance, did the pain start with an injury (such as a car accident, fall, or blow to the head) or after a specific activity or change (such as heavy lifting, a long drive, or a new pillow)?
- Where do you feel the pain? In the front, back, or side of the neck? Describe the location as precisely as possible, and whether you also have a headache or pain in the arm, chest, shoulder, or another area.
- How does the pain feel? Does it ache, stab, or burn? Have you had similar pain in other joints?

- Do you have any other symptoms along with the pain? Is there numbness, tingling, weakness, or stiffness in the neck, arms, shoulders, back, or other areas of the body?
- Is it worse or better at particular times of the day? Does it wake you up at night? Is it worse in the morning when you first arise?
- What eases the pain? Is it better when you rest, move around, or maintain a certain position?
- What makes it worse? Does it hurt more when your neck is in a certain position, when you eat, or when you do certain activities?
- How are you feeling otherwise? Do general symptoms of illness accompany your neck pain, such as fever, dizziness, nausea, blurry vision, difficulty concentrating, or depression?
- Do you have other chronic illnesses, such as arthritis, heart disease, cancer, or gastrointestinal problems? What is your current treatment?

Your doctor will need information not only about your present state, but also about past injuries and illnesses. Have you injured your neck before? How was your recovery? Previous illnesses and their treatment are sometimes relevant; for example, past radiation in the neck area may be linked to current pain.

How far should it go?

Your neck is the most flexible portion of your spine. If you have a full range of motion, you should be able to do the following:

- Touch your chin nearly to your chest. (This is called flexion, and it should allow movement of about 60 degrees.)
- Look almost straight up to the sky. (The term for this movement is extension, and it should allow you to tilt your head back about 70 degrees.)
- Rotate your head until it is even with your shoulders. (This is called rotation, and it allows you to turn your head about 80 degrees.)
- Tilt your head halfway to your shoulder. (This is a lateral bend, and it will let your head move about 45 degrees.)

Range of motion decreases somewhat with age, but ask your doctor to check on new or significant restrictions. Moving your neck through its complete range of motion daily can help prevent neck pain and help maintain a healthy range of motion.

Because your activities may provide clues about the cause of your pain, the doctor will also ask about your work, sports, other hobbies, and possible sources of physical and emotional stress.

Physical examination

Guided by your description of your pain, your doctor or other clinician will perform a general physical exam, with extra attention to things that might help explain your neck pain.

Posture. First, your doctor will observe your posture as you stand, sit, and walk. Your usual posture may be placing stress on particular muscles or neck structures. Conversely, neck pain may cause you to hold your head in a particular way.

Range of motion. Next, you may be asked to bend your neck forward, backward, and to the sides, and to turn your head as far as you can to the left and right. In addition, your doctor may check the passive range of motion in your neck and shoulders by moving them without your assistance. Range of motion diminishes somewhat as part of normal aging, but asymmetries, recent changes, or new abnormalities are important.

Neck muscles. He or she may look at and feel the strength and size of various muscles in the neck area, and press to identify tenderness in muscles or in the facet joints between the vertebrae. You should mention any pain or other sensations that occur in your neck or arms during any of these maneuvers.

Arms and hands. Your doctor will check your reflexes, muscle strength, and sensitivity to touch, such as a gentle pinprick or a light brush with a cotton swab at various points on your arms and hands. The spinal nerves that emerge from between the cervical vertebrae follow specific paths: pain or a distorted sensation along a track provides evidence that a particular nerve is being compressed, perhaps by a herniated disc or a bone spur.

Shoulders. During the examination, your shoulders will receive close attention, because shoulder and neck problems sometimes create similar symptoms.

During the general physical exam, your physician will also check for signs of medical conditions that sometimes cause neck pain, such as rheumatoid arthritis, heart disease, cancer, infection, or a thyroid condition. Even if an illness is unrelated to your neck pain, it may influence your doctor's choice of medication.

Imaging studies and other tests

There's a certain satisfaction when your physician displays a picture with an abnormality that seems to be at the root of your pain. Unfortunately, pinpointing the problem is not always that simple. While imaging techniques can provide some startlingly clear views of neck structures and are increasingly used (and many experts believe overused), there is often no clear relationship between what the imaging shows and what you feel. For example, the older you are, the more likely it is that imaging will show a disc abnormality or a narrowing of the spinal canal—even if your neck is pain-free. Imaging often reveals abnormalities that have nothing to do with the pain being investigated, and surgical correction of an unrelated abnormality has little chance of relieving your pain. For that reason, your physician should order imaging only when it is truly needed and take great care to ensure that your symptoms precisely match a correctable abnormality seen on an imaging study before considering surgery.

How do you know when imaging is truly needed? When pain is mild, the medical history and physical examination usually provide enough information without imaging. In other cases, some type of imaging may be appropriate—for example, if the pain is severe or doesn't respond to initial treatment, if there are signs of nerve damage, or if your doctor thinks you may have an infection, fracture, or tumor. When used and interpreted with caution, imaging can provide valuable details.

X-rays. Plain x-rays primarily show your bones and the spaces between them, as well as other calcium-containing tissues. The x-ray machine is positioned over the neck area to take pictures from the front and the side and, in some cases, while your neck is fully flexed and extended. X-rays of the neck are relatively imprecise. An x-ray may be falsely reassuring because many causes of neck pain don't involve specific abnormalities. On the other hand, x-rays of the cervical spine show abnormalities in more than one-third of adults with no neck symptoms.

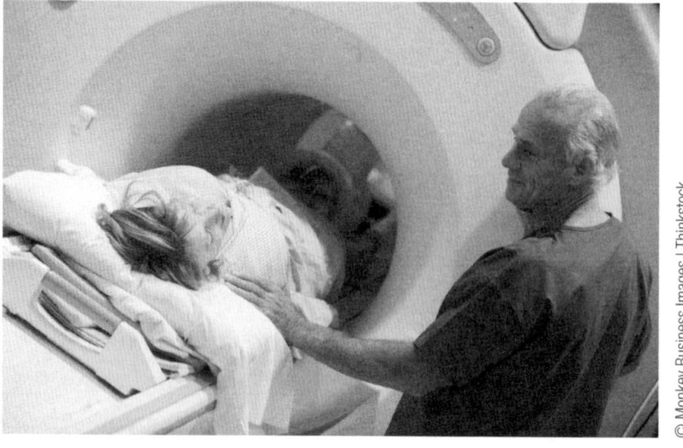

MRI is an excellent way to view the spinal cord, intervertebral discs, bones, and spinal nerves—and it doesn't expose you to radiation. But sometimes the damage it shows is unrelated to your pain.

Magnetic resonance imaging (MRI). MRI technology uses an intense magnetic field to create three-dimensional images from the minute electromagnetic waves emitted by body tissues. MRI is an excellent way to view the spinal cord, intervertebral discs, bones, and spinal nerves, and for this reason, it is increasingly used to evaluate neck pain. MRI has the added advantage of not exposing you to radiation. Your physician may recommend MRI if neck pain has not responded to treatment after several weeks or months, or sooner if you have severe pain, if you show symptoms of nerve damage, or if the doctor thinks you may have an infection or tumor. For the MRI procedure, you lie motionless in a large tube located in the center of a room-sized machine. The procedure lasts about half an hour. If you have a pacemaker or metal-containing implant, you cannot undergo MRI.

Computed tomography (CT). CT scans produce detailed images of bone and are used to detect a fracture or arthritis (even if regular x-rays are normal or inconclusive), but they are rarely used to evaluate neck pain because they are less effective than MRI for visualizing soft tissue such as nerves and discs. For a CT scan, you lie still for about 20 minutes on a table that slides into a tunnel-like scanner. A CT scan produces a detailed composite view of your neck. CT scans expose you to more radiation than a standard x-ray (see "Radiation safety," page 11). If your doctor thinks you may have an infection or tumor, a dye may be injected to highlight areas of inflammation on the CT scan.

Other tests

In addition, your doctor may order a variety of other tests that do not involve imaging.

Electrodiagnostic tests. Electrodiagnostic tests assess the function of muscles and nerves by measuring their electrical activity. They are used to obtain further information if your nerve function is abnormal in a way that suggests something is placing pressure on the spinal cord (myelopathy) or one of the nerve roots exiting the cervical spine (radiculopathy, or pinched nerve).

- **Electromyography (EMG)** uses fine needles that are inserted into your muscles to detect and record their electrical patterns at rest, in response to electrical stimulation of the nerves, and during voluntary muscle activity. Pressure on a nerve, nerve irritation, and other nerve and muscle problems can change the signals and the speed at which they are transmitted.
- **A nerve-conduction study** detects electrical signals through electrodes placed over a muscle or on an area of skin that receives signals from a specific nerve. The doctor uses a device to deliver a small electrical current to the skin near the nerve being tested. In response, the nerve fires and the resulting electrical signals are picked up by the electrodes and fed to a computer, which analyzes the timing and strength of the response. In most cases, a nerve-conduction study provides information that complements that obtained with EMG. It can be particularly helpful in determining the source of neck pain that radiates into the arm or is associated with weakness, numbness, or tingling.

Diagnostic nerve block. A diagnostic nerve block helps pinpoint the origin of neck pain. A local anesthetic is injected to deaden a specific nerve to see if that stops the pain. A diagnostic nerve block is usually reserved for unusual or confusing patterns of pain or pain that does not respond to treatment. Nerve blocks can also be used as a treatment.

Diagnostic facet joint injection. A diagnostic facet joint injection helps determine whether a facet joint is the source of your neck pain. A physician, usually an orthopedic surgeon or other pain specialist, injects a small amount of local anesthetic into the joint space; if that relieves your pain, it verifies that the facet joint is the source of your pain.

Laboratory tests. If needed, your physician may order blood tests and other laboratory tests to determine whether neck pain may be the result of a medical illness such as an infection, inflammatory arthritis, or cancer. If it's possible that you have meningitis, the doctor may recommend a lumbar puncture to remove a small sample of spinal fluid, which will then be tested for evidence of infection, tumor, or other causes of meningitis.

Radiation safety

X-ray machines and CT scanners emit radiation that enters your body and is captured by a camera to produce images. Many people are concerned when they hear that a test will expose them to radiation. In large amounts, radiation surely can cause cancer, scarring of tissues, reduced blood cell production, and other problems. The amount of radiation used in medical tests is generally too small to be harmful. For example, each of us is exposed to natural radiation on a daily basis, from such sources as cosmic rays from outer space. Exposure to radiation can increase with air travel and radioactive substances in the soil. A neck x-ray exposes us to an amount of radiation that is about the same as the radiation we are normally exposed to over 22 days. This is considered very little exposure. To get perspective, the average person is exposed to 360 millirems (mrem) of radiation per year, mostly from natural sources. A CT scan exposes us to 1,000 mrem, significantly more than a standard x-ray and natural exposure. Still, the upper limit of what is considered safe is 5,000 mrem in a single year.

Experts have raised concerns about the rapid increase in the use of medical imaging tests and caution people to make sure they have imaging scans only when needed.

Because radiation can cause birth defects in a fetus, women should tell their doctors whether they might be pregnant before having a medical test that uses radiation. If you are pregnant, your doctor will probably recommend waiting, unless he or she suspects a severe problem. For most cases of neck pain, imaging tests can wait.

Although radiation exposure to individuals is small, the cumulative exposure to technicians who perform the tests can be dangerous. That's why technicians wear lead shields or step outside the room to protect themselves. People who have been exposed to a lot of radiation because of their work should mention this to their doctors and have regular medical check-ups.

Common causes of neck pain

When your neck hurts, you want to know why. But be prepared for the possibility that your doctor may not be able to target a specific cause. You may be one of the many people who have pain but no clear abnormality. For many, the routine, daily demands on the structures of the neck result in pain. Lack of a diagnosable abnormality doesn't mean there is no solution, however. A number of treatments are available to help ease the pain.

Regardless of the cause, your goal is to relieve symptoms, to increase comfort, and to restore normal neck function. And treatments for different types of neck pain are often similar, no matter what the cause. Here are some of the most common disorders that can trigger neck pain, and an overview of treatment strategies for each. (For a more detailed description of treatment options, see the chapters that follow, including "Managing your pain," page 20; "Pain medications," page 33; "Complementary and alternative treatments," page 40; and "Surgery for neck pain," page 46.) Very rarely, neck pain may be a symptom of a serious condition that requires urgent care (see "When to seek immediate medical attention," page 6).

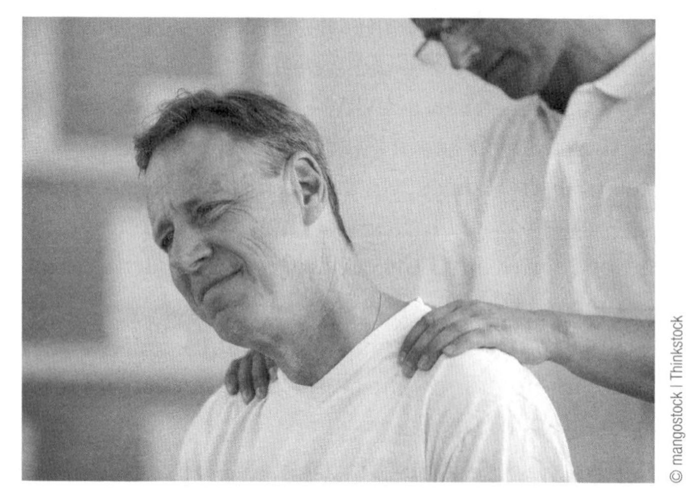

© mangostock | Thinkstock

Sprains and strains are by far the leading causes of neck pain, accounting for nearly 85% of cases. Most mild to moderate cases heal within a few weeks with simple treatments.

Neck strains and sprains

A strain is a muscle injury—the tissues overstretch or sustain microscopic tears as the result of repeated overuse or a single overexertion, such as hoisting a heavy suitcase. If the stretching and tears occur in a ligament, it is called a sprain.

Almost 85% of neck pain stems from either neck injury or stress and strain over the long term. Like other muscles, overworked neck muscles tend to become stiff and achy. In addition to overwork, neck strain or sprain can result from physical stress, poor posture, sleeping positions that don't support the neck in a healthy position (for example, sleeping on your stomach with your neck turned to the side), and injuries such as whiplash. Because a sprain or strain involves soft tissue, rather than bone, common imaging tests like x-rays won't reveal these injuries. Some doctors use the term "nonspecific neck pain" instead of strain or sprain.

➤ **Symptoms of neck strain or sprain.** The pain can range from mild to severe and often worsens with movement. In addition, a neck sprain or strain can cause stiffness, tightness in the upper back or shoulders, tension headaches, muscle spasms, or reduced ability to move the neck in one or more directions.

➤ **Treating strains and sprains.** Both strains and sprains need time to heal. In the meantime, conservative therapy—ice, pain medication, and heat—can help to alleviate discomfort. For the first one to two days, apply ice packs to the neck for up to 15 minutes out of every hour to numb the pain and reduce swelling. After two days, moist heat (applied with a warm, moist towel or in the shower or bath) can help to reduce pain. Over-the-counter pain relievers, including acetaminophen (Tylenol) and nonsteroidal anti-inflammatory drugs (NSAIDs) such as ibuprofen (Advil, Motrin), help relieve mild to moderate pain.

When pain strikes: An exercise to relieve neck pain

Here is a simple, gentle exercise to do when moderate neck pain first strikes. For severe pain, contact your health care provider immediately.

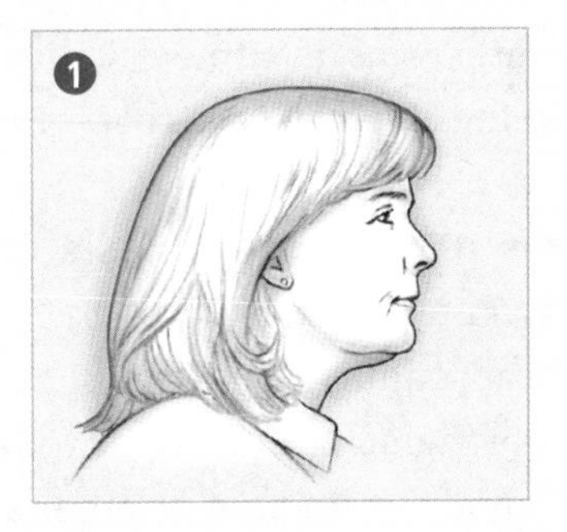

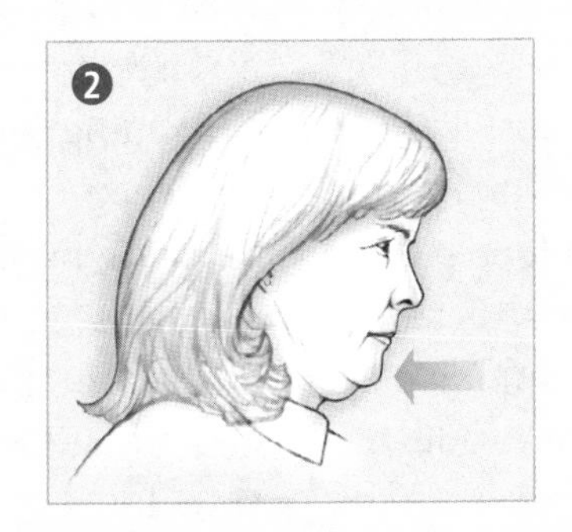

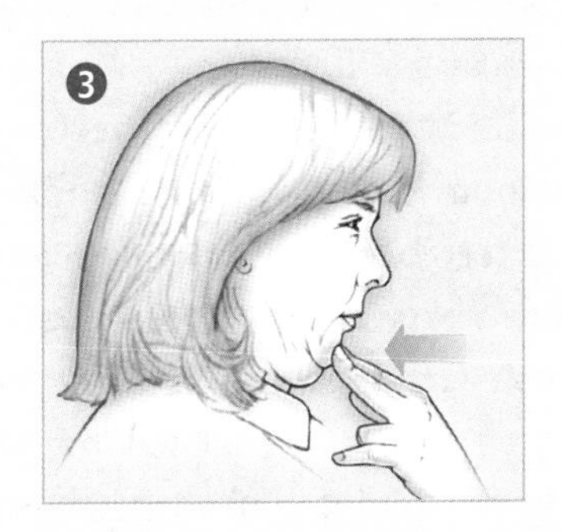

1. Sit in a neutral position, holding your head in a normal resting position.
2. Next, slowly glide your head backward, tucking your chin in until you have pulled your head and chin as far back as they will go. Keep your head level and do not tilt or nod your head. Pull in gently for three to five seconds, then release. Repeat 10 times.
3. For a stronger stretch, gently apply pressure to your chin with your fingers and release. Repeat every two hours as needed.

If this exercise increases your pain, try it lying down on your back. Tuck your chin in and make a double chin. Hold for a second or two and release (your head never leaves the pillow). If pain increases or you develop numbness or tingling, stop and contact your doctor.

You can use a soft neck collar sparingly to support your neck during periods when pain is intense. However, if overused, a neck collar can allow your muscles to become smaller and weaker (atrophy). So don't wear one for more than a few hours at a time or for more than one or two weeks at a stretch.

Once intense pain has subsided, use gentle stretching exercises to restore range of motion (see "Neck stretching," page 22). A physical therapy program that includes strength training exercises is fundamental to both treating neck pain and preventing future occurrences. Gently warming your neck with a heat pack before exercise may make it easier to do the exercises.

Most mild to moderate sprains and strains heal within two to three weeks with only these conservative treatments. For a more severe muscle spasm, your doctor might prescribe a muscle relaxant such as cyclobenzaprine (Flexeril). Most neck pain resulting from a sprain or strain will not require surgery.

If sprain or strain symptoms don't resolve with several weeks of care, your doctor may request x-rays or other diagnostic tests to look for other sources of neck pain, such as rheumatoid arthritis, bacterial infections, or a tumor.

Degenerative conditions

Over the years, age-related degeneration in the joints and discs of the neck may cause pain. Unfortunately, there are no specific measures you can take to prevent degenerative neck conditions other than trying to avoid neck injuries—for example, by wearing a seat belt or avoiding dangerous activities. Even exercise has not been shown to prevent or delay the onset of degenerative disc or joint disease in the cervical spine.

The initial, conservative treatments for pain from any of these degenerative conditions are the same as the initial treatments for neck pain stemming from sprains or strains. These treatments include ice packs, heat, pain relievers, gentle range-of-motion exercises, and when possible, stretching and strengthening exercises. Beyond that, treatments vary somewhat, based on which degenerative condition is involved.

Cervical osteoarthritis

Cervical osteoarthritis (also called degenerative arthritis, degenerative joint disease, or cervical spondylosis) results from the gradual breakdown of cartilage in the facet joints that connect the vertebrae.

Cartilage is connective tissue that cushions the ends of bones and reduces the friction between bones as joints move. As osteoarthritis progresses, the bones themselves grind together instead of gliding smoothly, causing pain and stiffness.

Over time, the vertebrae become distorted in shape, and bony overgrowths (osteophytes or, in common parlance, bone spurs) often develop, placing pressure on nerves that exit between the vertebrae. Cervical osteoarthritis is quite common among older adults as well as among people who have sustained a previous bone or joint injury in the neck.

➤ **Symptoms of cervical osteoarthritis.** The hallmark symptoms are pain radiating to the shoulders or between the shoulder blades; pain and stiffness that is worse first thing in the morning and at the end of the day; pain that eases with rest; and a crunching or grinding sound as you turn your head, caused by bone rubbing on bone.

➤ **Treating cervical osteoarthritis.** Occasional facet joint injections (in which a combination of a local anesthetic and an inflammation-reducing corticosteroid are injected into the facet joint) may help relieve pain. Surgery may be necessary if degenerative changes lead to compression of the spinal nerves or, even more seriously, to compression of the spinal cord or its blood vessels. The type of surgery performed will depend on the cause of the compression, which may include a herniated disc, bone spurs, or a narrowing of the spinal canal.

Spondylolisthesis and spondylolysis

Spondylolisthesis (also known as forward subluxation of the vertebra) occurs when one vertebra has slipped forward over another. It takes its name from the Greek words for spine (*spondyl-*) and slipping (*listhesis*). Although more commonly seen in the lower back, spondylolisthesis sometimes occurs in the neck, if aging discs and arthritic facet joints weaken the connections between vertebrae and allow an abnormal amount of movement to occur. Degenerative disease, such as arthritis, is the most common cause of spondylolisthesis in adults. Spondylolisthesis can also result from injury, repeated small fractures, or a birth defect of the spine.

Spondylolysis, on the other hand, is the fracture of a small area of bone (called the pars interarticularis) that connects the front and back of a vertebra on each side. Such tiny fractures may occur as the result of an injury, overuse (as in athletes), degenerative weakening (as in the elderly), or perhaps an inherited tendency.

➤ **Symptoms of spondylolisthesis and spondylolysis.** Key symptoms are pain, often radiating to the back of the head; stiffness; and numbness or weakness extending down one or both arms to the hands. Even in people who have no pain or other symptoms of spondylolisthesis or spondylolysis—particularly older people—an x-ray may show evidence of these conditions.

➤ **Treating spondylolisthesis and spondylolysis.** Physical therapy with a focus on stretching and strengthening exercises may help. Over-the-counter pain relievers are the first line of medication, and your doctor may prescribe a stronger, narcotic analgesic (such as codeine) for severe pain if necessary. Facet joint injections or injections of corticosteroids into the epidural space around the spinal nerves may also help. Surgery may be considered as a last resort. If spondylolisthesis has led to nerve compression, surgery is likely to involve both laminectomy (see page 46) and cervical spinal fusion (see page 47). The former creates more space for the nerves, and the latter stabilizes the cervical vertebrae, preventing further slippage and redevelopment of nerve compression. A fracture may be repaired with a bone graft taken from the pelvis.

Spinal stenosis

Degenerative changes in the spine can lead to spinal stenosis, a narrowing of the canal in which the spinal cord lies. This may result in a pinching of the spinal cord (see "Cervical myelopathy," page 16). Between 50,000 and 125,000 people in the United States report symptoms of spinal stenosis involving the neck. However, spinal stenosis is also visible on MRI scans of many older people without symptoms.

➤ **Symptoms of spinal stenosis.** Some people experience an aching pain aggravated by activity and relieved by bending forward, radiating pain down one or both arms or legs, arm or leg weakness, urinary frequency, or falls or other symptoms of instability. In some cases, no symptoms are apparent.

➤ **Treating spinal stenosis.** Conservative treatments, including a physical therapy program designed to strengthen abdominal and back muscles and preserve motion in the spine, may be enough to adequately relieve pain. If they do not, your doctor may prescribe stronger pain medications, or recommend facet joint injections or nerve root blocks. Alternative and complementary treatments, such as acupuncture, may also be worth a try (see "Complementary and alternative treatments," page 40).

Surgery is usually not considered for spinal stenosis until nonsurgical treatments have had a chance to work. However, it may be considered earlier if the spinal cord is being compressed, in order to avoid the possibility of permanent nerve damage. The aim of surgery is to relieve pressure on the spinal cord or nerves and restore the alignment of the spine. In one common procedure called laminectomy, the surgeon removes a part of the bone (the lamina) at the back of one or more vertebrae to create more space for the nerves. Parts of the facet joints may also be removed, along with any bone spurs or disc herniation. Someone with both stenosis and instability of the spine may also undergo spinal fusion.

Degenerative disc disease

Degenerative disc disease develops gradually as the shock-absorbing discs between the cervical vertebrae shrink and become less flexible over time. It can also occur in younger people who are highly active. The condition is common and often does not cause any pain or discomfort. In fact, degenerative disc disease can be seen on MRI scans of 25% to 40% of adults who are symptom-free. In others, however, this aging process can lead to a variety of symptoms. In reaction to the diminishing padding and stability formerly provided by the discs, the vertebrae may form bony overgrowths; these may cause no symptoms unless the spinal cord or nerves are compressed. If a disc's outer casing weakens or tears, the inner portion may bulge out (herniate) beyond the vertebra. A herniated disc can cause pain by spurring inflammation in the area or pushing on a nerve.

➤ **Symptoms of degenerative disc disease.** Symptoms include pain when rotating or bending the neck in the direction of a herniated disc; pain relieved by elevating the arm; and pain, numbness, or weakness in the arms because of pressure on a nerve. The severity of pain can vary widely from one person to the next.

➤ **Treating degenerative disc disease.** For degenerative disc disease, the initial approach is conservative: use of heat, pain-relieving medication, and gentle range-of-motion exercises. If surgery is necessary, the most common procedure for degenerative disc disease is anterior cervical discectomy and fusion. In this procedure, the diseased or damaged disc is removed, along with any bone spurs, through an incision in the front of the neck. This helps relieve pressure on the nerve roots or spinal cord. Selected vertebrae are then joined together with metal implants or bone grafts to restore stability.

Another option is the surgical implantation of an artificial disc (see page 48).

Nerve pain

The neck is packed with structures, including the spinal cord and peripheral nerves that lead to all parts of the body. When nerves in the neck are squeezed, pinched, or otherwise damaged, a variety of painful symptoms can result.

Pinched nerve (cervical radiculopathy)

Normally, nerves branch off the spinal cord through spaces between the vertebrae. If one of these exit spaces shrinks, it can squeeze the nerve root (the radicular nerve) and cause symptoms in the area served by the nerve. A number of problems can cause a pinched nerve, including a herniated disc, spinal stenosis, or degenerative disc disease. Age-related degenerative changes in the spine account for 70% to 90% of all cases.

➤ **Symptoms of pinched nerve.** When neck pain arises from compressed nerves, symptoms may include shooting pain in the neck, arms, shoulders, or upper back; pain that worsens with movement or coughing; numbness and tingling in the fingers; and difficulty coordinating fine movements, such as handwriting.

➤ **Treating a pinched nerve.** People with a pinched nerve have a good outlook for recovery. As a result, treatment almost always begins with conservative therapies. Your doctor will likely recommend an over-the-counter pain reliever. You will be advised to avoid activities that cause pain or discomfort and may be told to use a cervical collar for a brief period of time, as well as a cervical pillow while you sleep. Physical therapy, range-of-motion exercises, and strengthening exercises may help as well. If your pain is severe, your doctor may prescribe a short course of an oral corticosteroid. Anticonvulsant medications may also be used, and epidural glucocorticoid injections are sometimes given for persistent pain. Surgery is not usually considered unless the pain has not eased with six to eight weeks of conservative therapy, you experience increasing difficulty moving, or there is evidence of spinal cord compression. The most commonly used surgical procedure to relieve pressure on the spinal cord or radicular nerves is anterior cervical discectomy and fusion (see "Surgery for neck pain," page 46).

Cervical myelopathy

The term myelopathy refers to any disorder or disease of the spinal cord. Cervical myelopathy is a condition in which there is pressure on the cervical spinal cord or its blood vessels. Cervical myelopathy can be caused by narrowing of the spinal column that is present at birth (congenital). It can also be caused by spinal stenosis, bony overgrowths, a herniated disc protruding into the spinal canal, enlarged ligaments, or a combination of these problems. More rarely, cervical myelopathy may develop because of infection or a tumor.

➤ **Symptoms of cervical myelopathy.** Symptoms may mimic those of a pinched nerve. But while a pinched nerve tends to cause radiating symptoms in one arm, myelopathy may cause pain, weakness, or clumsiness in both arms or even in the legs. In some cases, it causes loss of bladder or bowel control. At its most severe, myelopathy causes permanent damage to the spinal cord that leads to disability. In some people, symptoms such as weakness and pain progress gradually; in others, symptoms worsen abruptly.

➤ **Treating cervical myelopathy.** Nonsurgical treatments include a cervical collar, avoidance of high-risk activities, and precautions to avoid whiplash, because minor neck injuries can cause an abrupt worsening of symptoms. Some physicians advise against exercise for this reason.

A variety of medications can also help control the pain. These include over-the-counter pain relievers, prescription opioid painkillers, muscle relaxants, or antidepressants, among others. However, these drugs tend to be more effective for peripheral neuropathy (such as diabetic neuropathy), where the nerve damage is close to the end of the nerve, rather than at the spinal cord, as it is with myelopathy.

Surgery is considered earlier for myelopathy than for a pinched nerve because of the potential for permanent damage to the spinal cord. A number of different surgical procedures may be used to treat cervical myelopathy, depending on the cause of compression to the spinal cord or its blood vessels. Anterior cervical discectomy, corpectomy (removal of the central portion of one or more vertebrae), laminectomy, and laminoplasty are surgical procedures that may be used alone or in combination to relieve pressure on the spinal cord or its blood vessels. (See "Surgery for neck pain," page 46, for more detailed explanations.)

Whiplash

Whiplash is the name for a group of symptoms and also for the typical accident that leads to them. Whiplash is also called a hyperextension or acceleration-deceleration injury, and while it is most commonly associated with car crashes, it can also occur in other situations, such as riding a roller coaster or getting punched in the face.

Whiplash injury can cause neck muscles to strain and ligaments to stretch or tear. Whiplash injury may also affect the spinal nerves, intervertebral discs, facet joints, or other components of the neck.

Whiplash damage to muscles and ligaments should heal within a few months. However, roughly one-third to one-half of people with whiplash do not recover fully, though their lingering symptoms tend to be mild and intermittent, and do not often interfere with work or daily activities. Of the one million people diagnosed with whiplash every year in the United

States, between 5% and 8% experience lingering pain and other ongoing symptoms severe enough to diminish their work capacity. If you are experiencing lasting symptoms, talk with your doctor, who may check for injuries to the facet joints and discs.

Since the late 1990s, scientists have gained a better understanding of what happens to the neck during a whiplash injury. Previously, it was believed that the initial impact jerks the head and neck back, and then they snap forward—thus whiplash. Now high-speed cameras and other instruments have shown that there is a critical moment or two before that back-and-forth. When your car is hit from behind, your torso is pushed forward by the force from the rear impact. As a result, your head moves both back and down. That motion bends the vertebrae in your upper neck back and those in the lower neck forward. Seen from the side, your neck momentarily looks like an S, as the upper and lower areas of your neck are unnaturally forced in different directions (see Figure 3, below). Researchers now believe that this "S phase" of whiplash is when injury is most likely to occur, as the muscles, ligaments, and joints strain to hold the vertebrae.

➤ **Symptoms of whiplash.** Symptoms go well beyond stiffness. They may include neck pain aggravated by movement; worsening pain in the days following an accident as tissues swell; shoulder pain; muscle spasms in the neck or upper shoulders; decreased range of motion; headache; tingling or weakness in the arms; and sometimes irritability, fatigue, sleep difficulties, or poor concentration.

Figure 3: Whiplash in action

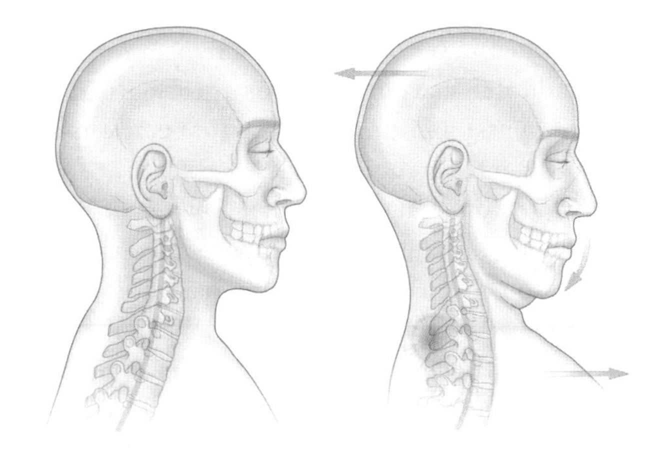

The force of a rear-end collision momentarily pushes the trunk forward and the chin down, forcing the cervical spine into an *S* shape and possibly damaging delicate structures.

➤ **Treating whiplash.** In the days immediately following a whiplash injury, ice packs will help control pain. Over-the-counter NSAIDs such as ibuprofen (Advil) or naproxen (Aleve) will also help relieve pain and control inflammation. It is important to begin gentle range-of-motion exercises and then isometric neck strengthening exercises as soon as you are able. Strong neck muscles help maintain proper head and neck posture, which in turn decreases the stress on muscles, discs, and vertebrae and gives damaged tissue the opportunity to mend. Heat packs can be used before exercising to relax joints and muscles. If over-the-counter NSAIDs do not adequately relieve pain, your doctor may prescribe a short course of a narcotic pain reliever or a muscle relaxant.

Facet joint injections may be used when more conservative approaches fail. Less commonly, radiofrequency neurotomy, a procedure that uses heat to block nerves from conducting pain signals, may be used to treat whiplash stemming from facet joint pain. Surgery is rarely used to treat whiplash, but may be done for individuals who continue to experience severe pain or disability after a reasonable period of nonsurgical treatment. Surgery is also more likely if the pain stems from one or two cervical discs, or if there is pressure on a nerve or on the spinal cord.

Recovery times for whiplash vary. One systematic review of 47 studies found that about half of adults with whiplash injury still had neck pain one year after the injury. One study showed that recovery time for victims of whiplash increased according to the number of visits to health care practitioners, especially for individuals who saw a chiropractor six or more times. The researchers suggested that "too much care" may actually increase a person's perception of disability, thereby increasing perceived recovery time. Another study found that the two most important predictors of pain at one year were the severity of pain at the time of the injury—and the presence of a compensation claim.

No matter how long you have been coping with whiplash-related symptoms, neck exercise may help.

In a 2016 Swedish study, people who were injured, on average, 22 months previously, were able to reduce their neck pain and disability by participating in supervised exercises. The exercises, taught in twice-weekly sessions with guidance for practicing at home, began gently and were progressively challenging. Meanwhile, while the exercisers improved, symptoms continued to worsen in people on a waiting list for care who received no exercise instruction.

General pain syndromes

Neck pain is a common symptom of disorders such as fibromyalgia and myofascial pain syndrome.

Fibromyalgia

Fibromyalgia is estimated to affect about five million adults in the United States. Of these, about 85% are women, most of them middle-aged, although the condition can also affect men and children. Although the cause of fibromyalgia is poorly understood, it may result from changes in the central nervous system that heighten a person's response to pain.

Figure 4: Tender points in fibromyalgia

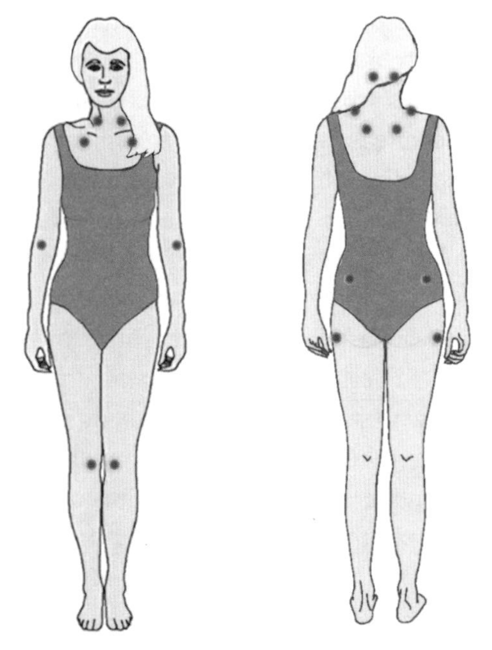

Areas of tissue that become painful when pressed, particularly in the locations shown, are called "tender points." They often develop in people with fibromyalgia.

➤ **Symptoms of fibromyalgia.** In general, the syndrome involves musculoskeletal pain, poor sleep, fatigue, and the presence of numerous points on the body that are tender to pressure (see Figure 4, below left). Longstanding neck pain is common. Fibromyalgia symptoms worsen with prolonged inactivity and withdrawal from activities.

➤ **Treating fibromyalgia.** Treatment focuses on relieving the underlying general pain syndrome rather than treating neck pain per se. Studies suggest that exercise, particularly aerobic exercise, can help relieve pain, increase tolerance of pressure on tender points, and improve well-being and physical function in individuals with fibromyalgia. There is also strong evidence that cognitive behavioral therapy, mindfulness meditation, and relaxation programs can help. Heat and massage can relieve musculoskeletal pain in the short term.

One medication used to treat seizures—pregabalin (Lyrica)—and two drugs that treat depression and neuropathy—milnacipran (Savella) and duloxetine (Cymbalta)—have been approved by the FDA to treat fibromyalgia. Other drugs commonly prescribed for fibromyalgia include another antiseizure medication, gabapentin (Neurontin), antidepressants such as amitriptyline (Elavil) and fluoxetine (Prozac), and the muscle relaxant cyclobenzaprine (Flexeril). Antidepressants, when prescribed at low doses, provide direct pain relief independent of their effect on mood.

Myofascial pain syndrome

Myofascial pain syndrome is a general pain syndrome that is related to fibromyalgia. The term "myofascial pain" indicates that it arises from problems in the muscles (*myo-*) and the bands of connective tissue (*fascia*) that wrap around muscles.

➤ **Symptoms of myofascial pain syndrome.** This condition is often diagnosed when people experience chronic pain and have hard, painful-to-touch trigger points along specific muscles. When the doctor presses a trigger point, the muscle may jump or twitch, and you may feel pain at that spot or another spot nearby that lies along the same nerve pathway (referred pain). However, neck pain attributed to myofascial pain syndrome often has no discernible trigger points in the neck. When a possible trigger point is identified, the doctor must ensure that the pain is not stemming from pressure on an underlying structure, such as a facet joint.

➤ **Treating myofascial pain syndrome.** As with fibromyalgia, treatment focuses on relieving the underlying pain syndrome. Individuals with myofascial pain syndrome may benefit from a physical therapy program that includes stretching and massage. Trigger point injections, inserted in and around trigger points, can also help to relieve muscle tension. These injections contain a small amount of anesthetic and may also contain corticosteroids to relieve pain and inflammation. NSAIDs help relieve muscle pain in some people with myofascial pain, but not others. Tricyclic antidepressants such as amitriptyline (Elavil), taken at low doses, can also help to relieve pain and improve sleep.

Other causes

Depending on your symptoms, and whether your neck pain was preceded by a trauma such as an accident, your doctor may order x-rays to check for a fracture. He or she may also order other tests to determine whether your pain stems from an underlying medical condition, such as one of the following:.

- Rheumatoid arthritis, an inflammatory disease that damages the lining of joints, usually attacks the hands and feet first, but neck joints may also be affected.
- Ankylosing spondylitis, another inflammatory disease, is more likely to be diagnosed because of pain in the lower back and pelvis, but as it continues to develop and worsen, it can also cause pain and stiffness in the neck.
- Bacterial infections of the bones or discs in the neck may cause neck pain; fortunately, these are relatively rare.
- A tumor, either originating in the neck area or spreading from another area of the body, may affect the bones or nearby nerves in the neck, causing pain.

Managing your pain

There is no magic bullet for neck pain, but there are plenty of ways to manage your condition so you can go about your daily life. The goal of treatment is threefold: to relieve pain, restore function, and reduce the risk of reinjury. You can use many of the pain-relieving strategies and exercises discussed in this section to ease flare-ups and prevent recurrences. A physical therapy program that emphasizes strength and stretching exercises, combined as needed with medication and relaxation therapies, often solves the problem or minimizes it to the point where you can resume most of your usual activities without pain. Some people also choose to combine these strategies with alternative or complementary therapies. Surgery, however, is not the treatment of choice for most kinds of neck pain.

Choosing a physical therapist

When choosing a physical therapist, check to make sure he or she is licensed by the state. A therapist must have a graduate degree from an accredited physical therapy program in order to be licensed. If you choose to see a physical therapist assistant, he or she should be supervised by a licensed physical therapist.

You may also want to look for a physical therapist who participates with your insurance company or will submit claims on your behalf to your insurance company. You can also ask your insurance company for a list of preferred providers who are covered. You may need a referral from your primary care physician before you see a physical therapist.

Another factor to consider is where the therapist practices. Depending on your preference, you can choose a therapist who practices in a hospital, private practice, outpatient clinic, rehabilitation facility, or a number of other settings. Some physical therapists make home visits.

The American Physical Therapy Association (APTA) has a searchable database of APTA members across the country on its website, www.apta.org.

QuickTip | **Heat and cold packs may be eligible for coverage if you have a medical Flexible Spending Account through your employer, making the income spent to cover these expenses tax-free.**

Initial steps

If the pain is severe or sharp, you will need to rest your neck and also use ice, heat, or both. (In some cases, though, you may need medical help; see "When to seek immediate medical attention," page 6.)

Rest. Unless you have sustained a significant injury, such as a neck fracture or ruptured disc, total or prolonged bed rest is not recommended for neck pain. However, for many conditions, specific rest techniques have an important role to play in reducing pain and preventing further damage to injured structures.

First, avoid quick movements, positions that hurt, and whatever activity you think caused the pain. Second, rest with your neck in a healthy position. Lying down for 20 to 30 minutes with your neck supported in a neutral position (not twisted) gives you a break from supporting the weight of your head (see "Resting technique," page 21).

In some cases, a cervical collar may help rest your neck muscles and protect damaged tissues from painful movements. If this is the case, your physician may prescribe one made of foam or plastic and fastened with Velcro, to hold your neck upright. Prolonged or constant use of such collars is generally no longer advised because it limits range of motion and may cause neck muscles to weaken (though constant use may be temporarily needed after surgery). If a cervical collar is prescribed, wear it as necessary for a week or so following your injury, removing it several times a day to exercise your neck, unless your doctor instructs you otherwise. Wear the collar in bed if it helps you sleep. As soon as you are able, reduce your use of the collar until you can eliminate it entirely. Over time, people with neck injuries recover more fully if they begin exercising soon after an injury.

Cold and heat. Cold numbs pain and reduces swelling by constricting blood vessels and dampening the body's inflammatory reaction. You can apply cold to an injured neck by wrapping an ice pack (or even a bag of frozen peas) in a cloth and applying it for 15 to 20 minutes out of every hour. To prevent frostbite, do not apply ice directly to the skin for more than a minute.

Heat, applied for about 15 minutes at a time, is a good way to reduce pain and stiffness and relieve muscle spasms. You can apply a heat pack directly to the sore or tense areas of your neck. You can purchase heat packs and moist/dry heating pads, but a homemade heat pack works just as well. Heat a damp folded towel in a microwave oven (usually for about 10 to 60 seconds, depending on the oven and the towel's thickness). Avoid overheating the towel, which can injure your skin. Therapists often recommend a warm shower or bath before exercising to relax joints and muscles.

After an injury, use ice for a maximum of 15 to 20 minutes an hour for the first 24 to 48 hours. After that, you can alternate ice and heat or use either ice or heat alone. Ice increases stiffness; you may find it beneficial to use warmth before stretching and other exercise, following with ice afterward to minimize swelling.

Although heat and cold have long been used to manage neck pain and many people report that these measures help, the scientific evidence of their benefit is not conclusive.

Resting technique

Lie on your back, using a pillow under your knees to help your back relax. Support the curve of your neck from the base upward, using a rolled-up towel, foam cylinder, or cervical pillow specially designed to support the neck. When you get up, turn onto your side and use your hands to push yourself to a sitting position; this avoids use of your neck muscles.

Physical therapy

If you have neck pain, you may benefit from working with a physical therapist, who can create an individualized treatment program for you, based on your specific needs and goals. This program can help reduce or eliminate pain, improve or restore mobility and function, and prevent disability.

Physical therapy for neck pain can be divided into two categories: active and passive therapies—that is, things the therapist teaches you to do for yourself and things he or she does for you. Because active therapeutic exercise has taken center stage as the best way to speed recovery, a physical therapy session is likely to focus on teaching you a set of appropriate exercises tailored to your specific neck problem; these exercises not only stretch tight areas and build strength, but also teach you proper body mechanics to heal your neck and reduce the risk of reinjury. (See "Gentle exercises for neck pain," page 22, for examples of some types of exercises your physical therapist might teach you. Our exercises are gentle ones that you can learn and do on your own.)

The session may also include one or more of the following passive pain-relieving interventions, but even these are done to allow you to participate in an exercise program and begin rehabilitating your neck.

Ultrasound. Therapeutic ultrasound (also called ultrasound diathermy) converts sound waves outside the range of human hearing into heat that penetrates into deep tissues. It is used to treat several conditions that can affect the neck, including muscle pain and degenerative arthritis.

If you receive ultrasound, the therapist will first spread a gel over the affected area to reduce friction. The ultrasound is delivered through a wand rubbed gently over the area for several minutes; you may feel a tingling sensation. Ultrasound treatments are usually administered repeatedly over a number of weeks. Ultrasound is safe for most people; however, people with certain types of implanted devices, such as a defibrillator or a neurostimulation device, should not undergo therapeutic ultrasound on the neck, even if the device is turned off. As with other heat treatments, no controlled trials have provided solid evidence for or against the benefit of ultrasound in neck pain.

Gentle exercises for neck pain

Perform these movements to the point where you feel a slight stretch but no pain. **Note:** While these exercises are fine for most people with neck problems, do not do them if you have a fracture or a recent, significant neck injury, or when movement exacerbates the pain. Check with your doctor if you've had a recent neck trauma, or you're not sure you should exercise your neck.

Neck stretching

These stretches help relieve tight neck muscles. At the same time, they reduce compression of the vertebrae caused by such tension, and they help maintain or extend the neck's range of motion.

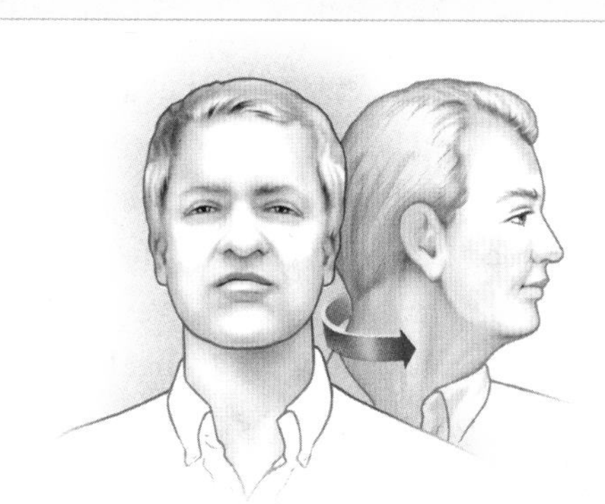

Rotation range-of-motion

Start by facing forward. Turn your head slowly to one side. Hold three seconds and return to the original position. Turn your head slowly to the other side. Hold three seconds and return to the original position. Repeat 10 times.

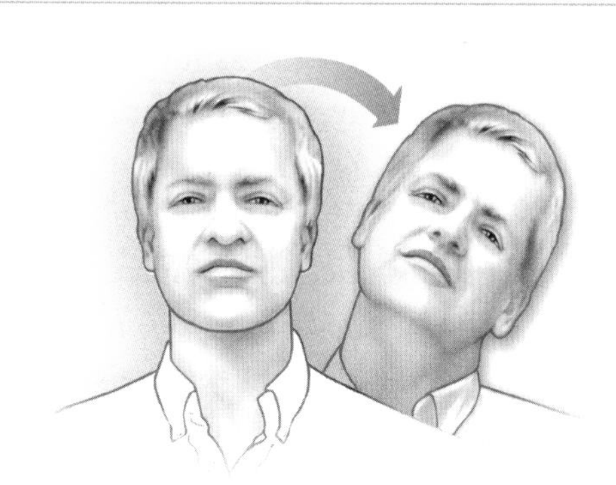

Side bending range-of-motion

Face forward and let your head bend slowly to the side. Hold three seconds and repeat to the other side. Repeat 10 times. Do this exercise slowly and gently. For an additional stretch, when your head is bent to the side, let it roll slowly forward about 45 degrees and hold it there for three seconds.

Acknowledgement: Physical therapists Nancy Capparelli and Tina Nebhnani of Beth Israel Deaconess Medical Center in Boston helped design this program.

Neck strengthening

Strengthening the muscles surrounding the cervical spine alleviates some of the pressure on the facet joints. It also helps maintain proper alignment of the spine, which in turn reduces muscle strain on the surrounding areas.

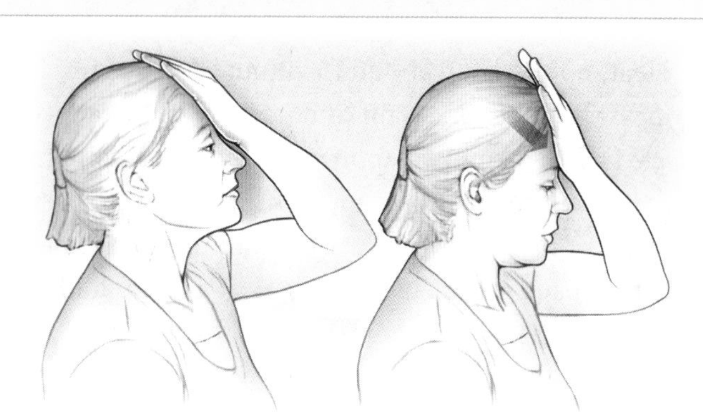

Front neck muscles:

This exercise can be done in a sitting position—at the office, for example—or lying down with your knees bent and feet flat on the floor. Place your palm on your forehead and press gently as you try to bring your chin to your chest; your neck muscles will tighten without your head moving. Hold for a count of three to five seconds. Repeat 10 times, twice daily.

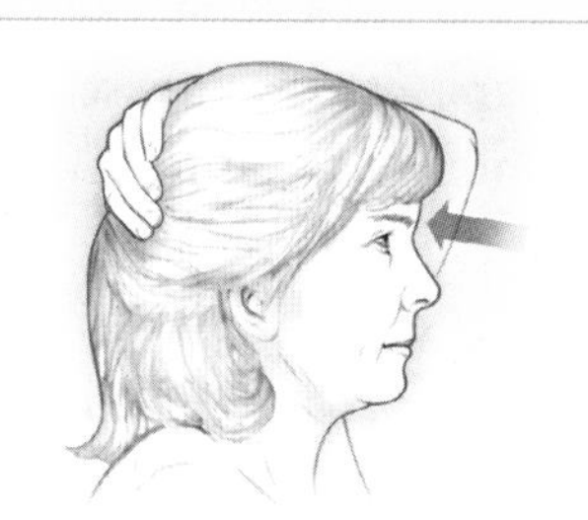

Rear neck muscles:

Place one or both hands behind your head and use them to resist as you press your head backward. Hold for a count of three to five. Repeat 10 times, twice daily.

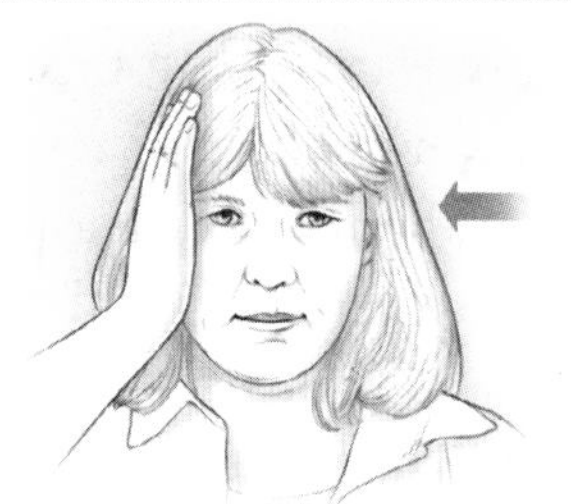

Side neck muscles:

Place your right palm on the right side of your head, using it to resist as you try to bend your right ear toward your shoulder. Hold for a count of 10. Repeat on the left.

Rotation muscles (not shown):

Place your right hand on the right side of your head. Try to rotate your head to the right, resisting with your hand. Hold for a count of three to five. Repeat on the left. Repeat 10 times.

Shoulder strengthening

Strengthening the shoulder muscles in addition to the neck muscles also helps to improve neck pain in the short and long term, perhaps by reducing pressure on the joints and nerves in the neck.

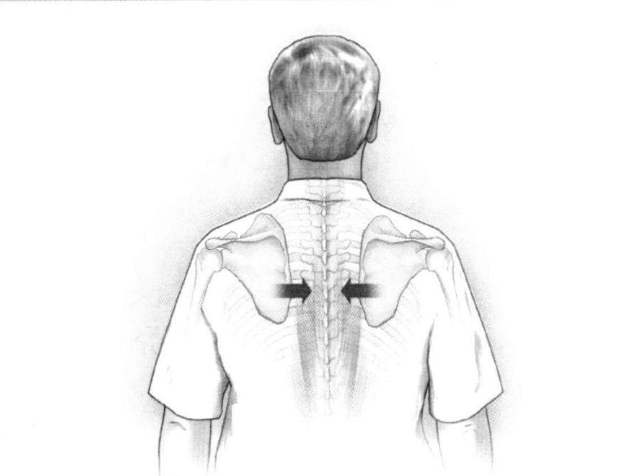

Shoulder blade retractions

Stand up straight with your arms at your sides. Squeeze your shoulder blades together for a count of four and release. Repeat 10 times.

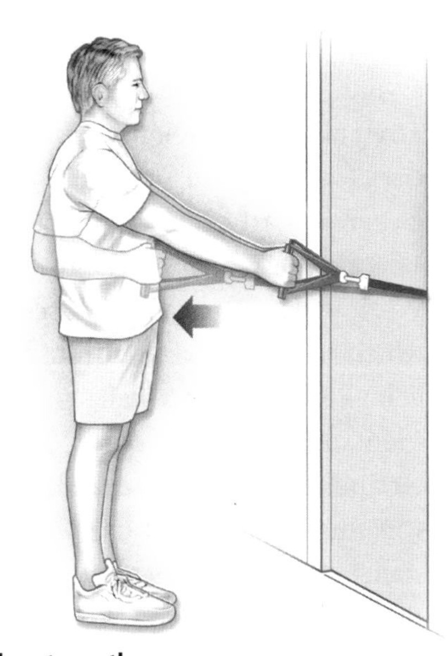

Shoulder strengthener

Secure an elastic exercise band (available at sports and fitness stores) to a sturdy post or railing at waist level. With arms extended, hold the ends of the elastic taut. Pull back slowly, bending your elbows at waist level and squeezing your shoulder blades together. Return slowly to the starting position. Perform three sets of 10 repetitions. Rest one minute between sets.

Transcutaneous electrical nerve stimulation (TENS). In this therapy, small adhesive electrodes are placed strategically on your skin at or near the sites of pain or dysfunction. These electrodes transmit an electrical current of very low voltage to underlying tissues, so you feel tingling rather than pain. TENS does not increase muscle tension. TENS is usually applied in a health care setting, but small home units—with a power source about the size of a cellphone—are available.

You can use TENS for 20 to 60 minutes at a time. It does not have a direct impact on the underlying cause of pain, but by relieving the symptoms it may help you participate in an exercise program or other therapy. TENS is considered safe; however, if you have a pacemaker, consult your cardiologist before using TENS. In addition, TENS should not be applied to the front of the neck because of the risk of stimulating the vagus nerve, which could slow down your heart.

Studies on the effectiveness of TENS have had mixed results. An analysis of several studies on TENS was unable to draw any conclusions because of the poor quality of most of the studies. But one randomized trial found that people with chronic neck pain who were treated with TENS twice a week for six weeks had significant improvement in disability, pain, and isometric neck strength six months after treatment, compared with those in the control group. Exercise had a similar effect as treatment with TENS.

Traction. To apply traction, a physical therapist uses hands, weights, or specialized equipment to create a sustained pull on the neck. Traction may be used to reduce spasms by stretching the muscles, or to create more space between the vertebrae, thereby relieving pinched nerves. Traction may be applied for 20 to 30 minutes at a time and repeated several times a day or only once a week. In a 2014 study, researchers treated 86 people with neck pain and symptoms of irritated nerves in the neck region. All the participants received neck exercises to do at home, but in addition, one-third received a home over-the-door traction unit, while another third received traction from a physical therapist. After four weeks, all the participants felt better, but only those who received manual traction from a physical therapist maintained significant improvement at six months and one year, achieving a 20% reduction in disability.

Your insurer may cover an over-the-door home traction device if your doctor prescribes it. Different types of traction devices, capable of applying more force, may be covered if over-the-door traction hasn't helped and you have gained relief in physical therapy sessions using the alternative devices.

Inversion therapy is a form of traction in which an individual hangs upside down, with the aid of gravity boots, inversion tables, or other devices. The idea is that hanging upside down reverses the effects of gravity and increases the space between vertebrae. In truth, inversion therapy does not do either of these things, although it may temporarily extend the spine and briefly relieve muscle spasm. Inversion therapy does have potential side effects, which include a temporary worsening of high blood pressure (hypertension) and some back problems. For now, the unproven benefits don't outweigh the potential risks.

Exercise

There is mounting scientific evidence that specific exercises—and physical activity in general—help people break longstanding cycles of neck pain and heal more quickly after neck injury. After a whiplash injury, for example, people heal sooner and are less likely to develop chronic pain if they start gentle exercise as soon as possible. In easing chronic neck pain, the results from controlled studies are mixed, but all endorse staying active in some form.

One review of the research found evidence that exercise programs to stretch and strengthen either the neck alone or the neck plus the shoulders and trunk region improve pain in the short and long term compared with control treatment.

The same review did not find clear evidence that strengthening exercises alone can provide pain relief for chronic neck pain. However, one of the most frequently cited studies on the topic, published in *The Journal of the American Medical Association*, suggests that neck strengthening exercises by themselves are highly effective. The yearlong study looked at female office workers with chronic nonspecific neck pain who participated in different exercise treatments. The women who used neck strengthening exercises reported less neck pain than the women who stretched and did aerobics. (The study did not consider a combination of neck-focused strengthening and stretching.) Those who took part in even more intensive strength training, using elastic bands to provide resistance during strengthening exercises, did best of all. Both of the groups who did neck exercises had less pain and disability and better neck strength and range of motion than those who exercised without specific attention to rehabilitating neck muscles.

Despite this growing body of evidence, fewer than half of people who see a health professional for chronic neck or back pain are prescribed exercise as part of their treatment plan.

Therapeutic exercise often begins under the direction of a physician, physical therapist, or trainer who can create an individualized exercise program based on your pain severity, limitation of movement, and present strength. The program should have clearly stated goals and should include stretching and strengthening exercises, as well as exercises to improve how you use your neck muscles. (For some simple examples of stretching and strengthening moves, see "Gentle exercises for neck pain," page 22.)

Isometric exercises are often emphasized early in rehabilitation because muscle use is controlled and the risk of injury is low. Isometrics are muscle-building exercises in which you contract your muscles against resistance (such as a weight or a wall) but there is no larger movement. A good example is putting your palms together and pressing. In the neck strengthening exercises in this section, you use your hands to provide resistance. It's important to keep your head upright, in the neutral position. Work against the resistance for up to three to five seconds at a time, then ease off the pressure and relax.

Ideally, if you are working with a therapist, he or she will guide you through appropriate exercises, motivating you to work hard enough to see results but not induce further injury. At some point, you will be given exercises to do at home. Your therapist is likely to prescribe exercises for you to do between sessions, and your insurance may only cover a limited number of visits to a health professional. Before you exercise independently, make sure you understand which exercises to do and how to do them safely. Ask for written instructions and illustrations if you are still unsure.

Guidelines for exercise

When exercising on your own, follow these safety guidelines:

- Warm up with a gentle aerobic activity, such as walking or riding an exercise bike, before exercising the neck. You can also use a heating pad or warm compress to warm your neck up before exercise.
- Perform exercises slowly and carefully.
- Never exercise to a point that results in pain. If exercise causes moderate or severe pain, stop, apply ice, and don't repeat the exercise until you consult a health professional.
- If you're using weights, avoid doing too much too soon. Start with the minimal amount of weight and build up gradually.
- Apply ice after a workout as needed, especially when you first begin, to minimize swelling and discomfort.

Preventing further neck pain

As with so many things, when it comes to neck pain, an ounce of prevention may be worth a pound of cure. It's true that some causes of neck pain, such as age-related wear and tear, are not under your control. On the other hand, there are many things you can do to minimize your risk of recurring neck pain.

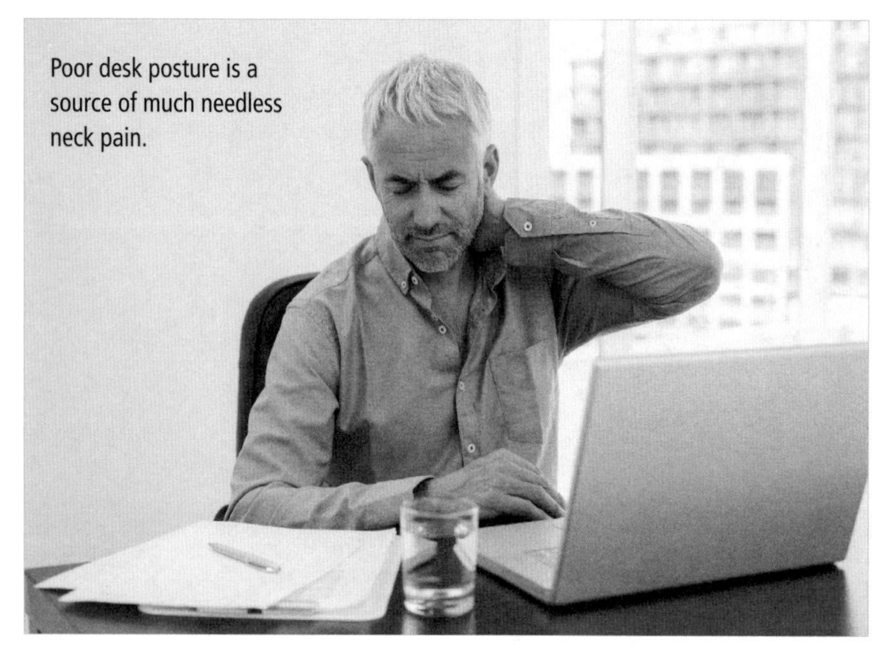

Poor desk posture is a source of much needless neck pain.

For example, one review that looked at risk factors for neck pain found an unexpected correlation between smoking and neck pain, for reasons that remain unclear. Not all of the studies found smoking to be a factor, but the possibility that smoking might contribute to neck pain provides extra incentive to kick the habit.

Other steps are simple and rely upon common sense: go about your daily activities placing as little stress and strain on your neck as possible. This includes everything from creating a workspace that encourages healthy posture and body mechanics to selecting a pillow that supports the natural curve of your neck. You can also make neck-friendly modifications to your favorite sports and leisure activities. Though it may take some getting used to, healthy neck posture now can help prevent future neck pain.

Ergonomics: Moving and sitting safely

Without knowing it, you may be encouraging neck pain by the way you perform everyday activities. Ergonomics is the field that translates what is known about physical and psychological health into specific advice for arranging your home and workplace so you can learn to do tasks safely and efficiently. You can start with the advice offered in this section. If you want more individual advice, seek help from a physical or occupational therapist who can assess your posture and body mechanics and help you learn to do your work, home chores, and recreational activities without straining your neck.

How you carry yourself can invite neck pain or help keep it at bay. In general, try to keep your neck in a neutral position, which means your head balances directly over your spine and is not leaning forward or cocked to one side. That's because your neck's principal job is to support your head, and your head weighs a lot—about 10 to 12 pounds. You can handle the weight well when your head is slightly tilted back—a position that best distributes its weight over the spine. However, the average person tilts his or her head forward slightly, which has the effect of putting more weight on the neck. A recent study calculated that flexing your head 15 degrees forward—a common position used to scan a cellphone, for instance—has the effect of magnifying its weight to 27 pounds. Lowering your head farther adds more effective weight. The more weight you put on your neck, the more likely you are to have neck pain.

Here are some hints for achieving a healthy neck posture in common activities.

At the computer or desk. When working at your computer or at a desk, keep your head balanced directly over your spine as much as possible. That means setting your chair height so both your feet can rest on the ground, and sitting with your buttocks far back in your chair, using a small pillow to support your lower back if needed (see Figure 5, below). Properly adjusting the keyboard and monitor may be difficult or impossible with a laptop, notebook, or tablet computer. You can plug in a separate, full-size keyboard to help you achieve better positioning. If that's not an option, a 2012 Harvard study showed that placing your laptop or notebook computer on a desk of standard height and propping it to about a 12% incline (a one-inch book or ring binder should do the trick) keeps your head and neck in a healthier position. The downside is that it does place slightly more stress on your wrists.

No matter how perfect your office-chair posture, it's important to get up and move around every half-hour, as prolonged sitting has been linked to worsening of neck pain and other health problems. If you tend to get lost in your work,

Figure 5: Desk posture

Take control of your body posture by setting up your chair, desk, and computer to encourage healthy neck and back positioning.

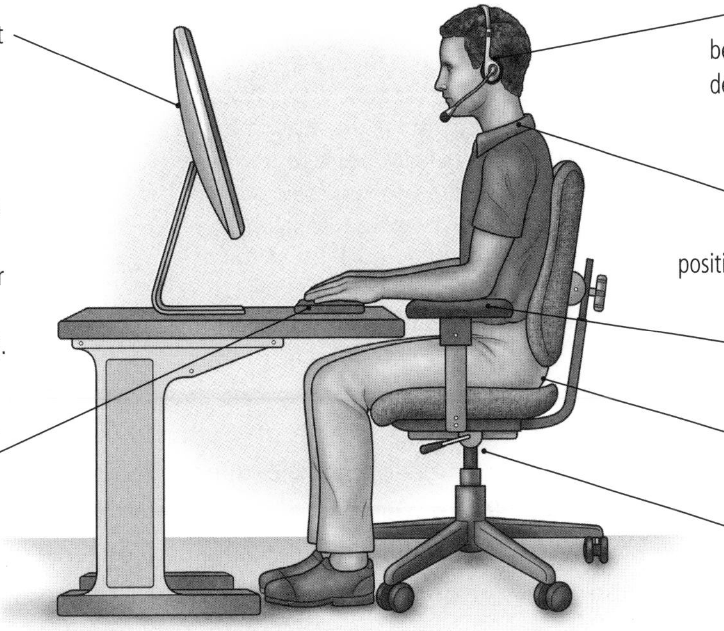

The flexible workstation

If your job requires you to work at a desk, you probably spend about half of your day sitting, and that's a problem. Prolonged sitting has recently emerged as a risk factor for neck pain and other serious health problems, including type 2 diabetes, obesity, heart disease, cancer, and even premature death. The workplace has therefore become a target for public health initiatives aimed at reducing time spent sitting.

Making their way into office spaces are several types of workstations that encourage you to stand. The treadmill desk allows workers to not only stand but also walk slowly while performing desk-related tasks. It has drawn considerable attention as its popularity has grown, with media reports of many who have been able to lose weight and reduce their risk factors for disease. No studies have yet looked at its effect on neck or back pain. However, it's well established that reducing the amount of time spent sitting can be very helpful in improving neck pain, so it's not unreasonable to try.

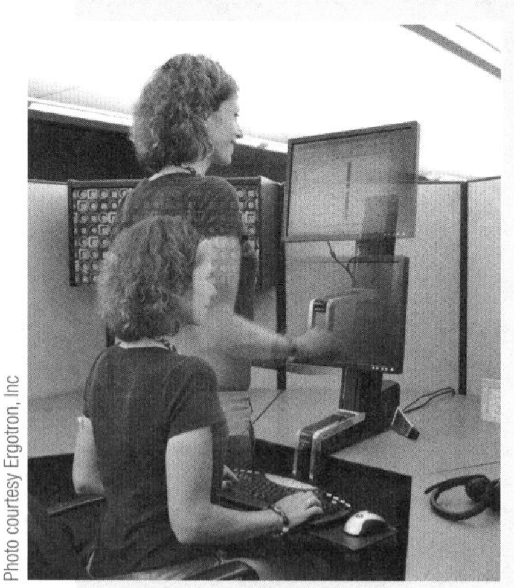

Photo courtesy Ergotron, Inc

Another type of desk, which allows you to adjust the height of your computer, enables you to switch between a sitting position and a standing position throughout the day (see photo, at left)—and there is at least preliminary evidence it may help neck pain. A small study, published in *Preventing Chronic Disease*, found that workers who voluntarily spent about an hour a day standing in these sit-stand workstations reduced their neck and upper back pain by 54%. They also felt happier, had more energy, and reported less stress. The study was performed over three months at a nonprofit health care firm, HealthPartners in Minneapolis. Participants included 34 employees in the health promotions division of that company who have sedentary desk jobs. Of this group, 24 employees used one of two types of sit-stand devices developed by Ergotron, Inc., a sponsor of the study. With these devices, monitors, keyboards, and a platform to hold documents can be elevated or lowered to an appropriate height so that the workers could change positions from sitting to standing at their discretion. The other 10 employees, who served as the comparison group, sat at their desks as usual. The study not only found improvement in pain, but also reported that these improvements diminished two weeks after the devices were removed. Larger studies are needed to confirm the results.

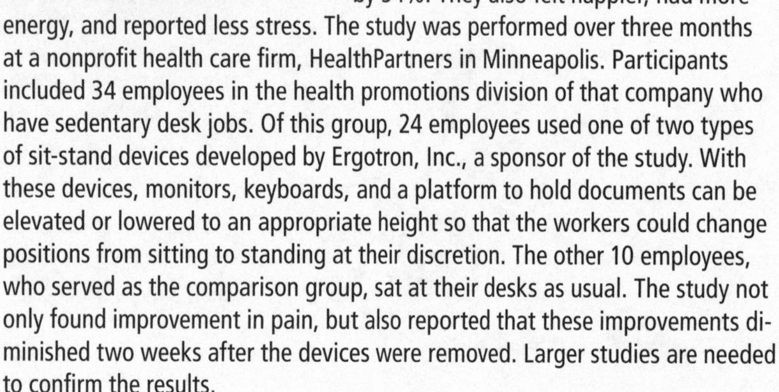

program your computer to flash a reminder, or set an alarm on your smartphone. Stretching can help, too. Shrug your shoulders up and down or lean your head to each side while pulling the opposite shoulder down.

Telephone use. If you spend a lot of time on the phone, try to avoid leaning your head to one side. This is also important when you use a cellphone and aren't sitting at your desk while you speak. A headset, earbuds, or speakerphone are good options to help keep your head in a neutral position for hands-free talking. Headsets are available for both your desk phone and cellphone.

Reading or writing at your desk. When reading, sit up straight and hold the document or book up so you don't need to bend over. Use your armrests to help support it, or use a document holder that props the material upright if you are reading or typing from a written document at your desk. For writing, adjust the chair and desk (blocks may help) so you needn't bend over. Paper can also be held on a slant board that raises it slightly off the desk and keeps it at a comfortable angle.

Reading at home. If you are sitting in a chair, try to maintain an upright posture. Hold the book so that you don't have to lean down or forward to see it. A pillow on your lap may help. If you must read in bed, sit up straight or use a specially designed wedge pillow. Or lie on your side with your neck straight and hold the book in front of you.

Wearing progressive lenses. The bottom portion of progressive lenses or bifocals is corrected for close-up vision. As a result, some people find that they need to bend their heads to see the ground clearly while walking or climbing stairs.

Over time, your brain generally learns to compensate, but if you find yourself staring down a lot while you walk, consider purchasing a pair of "walking glasses" that has your distance prescription but no bifocal reading lens. Another option is to purchase glasses with a different prescription for each eye—one for distance, one for close work.

In addition, if you spend a lot of time in mid-range activities, such as working on the computer or playing the piano, you may want to invest in a pair of glasses with an intermediate prescription between your reading and distance prescriptions. Most progressive lenses have a narrow mid-range—and bifocals don't have one at all—so you can strain your neck trying to see in focus. "Computer glasses" can help relieve not only neck strain, but also eye strain. Alternately, you may be able to move your monitor and adjust the font size so you can read the screen while looking through the upper portion of your glasses.

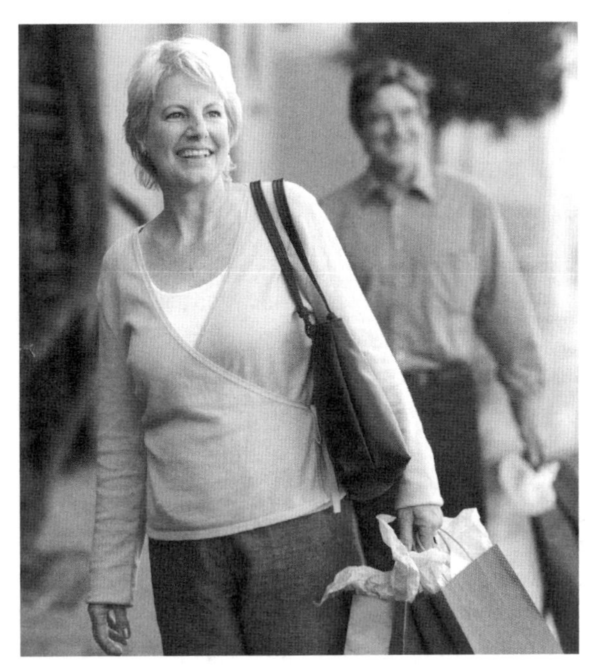

If you use a shoulder bag, transfer it from one side to the other every few minutes as you walk. A backpack that puts weight on the hips is the best choice for carrying objects.

Choosing the right shoes. Avoid high heels, which change the alignment of your body from the ground up, characteristically ending in a head-thrust-forward position that stresses neck muscles. This may be one reason women have neck pain more than men do.

Carrying a bag. Choose a lightweight purse or backpack, and don't overload it. Don't sling a backpack over one shoulder. Try switching to a fanny pack or a backpack designed to put weight on the hips instead of just the upper back. With heavier loads, use a wheeled pack or briefcase. If you must hoist a purse on your shoulder, alternate which shoulder you use.

Driving. Your posture is a factor in whether a crash will cause whiplash. To work properly, your headrest should be high enough and close enough to catch your head in a rear-end collision. Position the seat so you can sit up straight with your head no more than two to four inches in front of the headrest. Adjust the headrest so its upper edge is level with the top of your head: the back curve of your skull should meet the cushion of the headrest. If you drive long distances, periodic breaks can help to reduce or prevent neck strain.

Working overhead. Changing a light bulb, painting a ceiling, or even gazing at the stars in the night sky can invite neck strain and injury, particularly if you are reaching, twisting, or standing at an awkward angle. Use a ladder or scaffolding, and move it often in order to stay as close to your work as possible. Invest in long-handled tools. Take breaks to stretch, and switch back and forth between overhead tasks and those requiring a different position and motion.

Lifting. Improper lifting techniques put stress on the neck as well as the lower back. Bend your hips and knees instead of your back. Keep the object close to you while straightening your legs. When lifting something over your head, don't tilt your neck back. Strengthen your arms to make proper lifting easier.

Watching TV. Sit far enough from a TV or movie screen that you can watch without tilting your head back. Don't sit off to the side, which forces you to turn your neck for long periods.

Athletics and your neck

Staying physically fit is generally good for your neck. Any exercise that builds core strength,

Walk this way

Walking comes so naturally to most of us that we may not even give a second thought to proper walking technique. But an improper gait can lead to a host of complaints, including a stiff neck.

The good news is that it's possible to correct decades of ingrained walking habits with a little work. In fact, even if you don't think your gait is ungainly, you might benefit from the following tips:

- **Look ahead.** Lift up from the top of your head. Don't tuck your chin or look at the ground, but train your sights 10 to 20 feet ahead of you. If you need to check the ground to avoid obstacles, lower your eyes, not your head. An erect head reduces the likelihood of neck pain.
- **Stretch your spine.** Your shoulders should be level and square, neither thrust back nor slumped forward. Tuck your buttocks in. When your body is in alignment, you should be able to draw an imaginary straight line from your ear to your shoulder, hip, knee, and ankle when viewed from the side.
- **Bend your arms.** Flex your elbows at close to 90-degree angles and let your arms swing at waist level. Your fingers should be curled, but not clenched in a fist.
- **Swivel your hips.** A slight pivot at the hip can add power to your stride.
- **Flex your feet.** Come down on your heel; lift up off your toes. A person walking behind you should be able to see the sole of your shoe as you walk.
- **Take measured steps.** Too long a stride throws you off balance. Concentrate on taking shorter steps, but more of them.
- **Share your load.** Any load on the back or shoulders is likely to affect posture by thrusting the trunk forward. A backpack, which distributes weight evenly, is the best choice for carrying objects. If you use a shoulder bag, transfer it from one side to the other every few minutes as you walk.

for example, tends to help by encouraging better posture, which means that the head is balanced properly over the neck, avoiding strain. Pilates is a form of exercise that's known for helping develop core muscles. Harvard Medical School also has two Special Health Reports on building core strength (see "Resources," page 50).

But not all sports and exercises are equally easy on the neck. Bicycling, for example, is an excellent, low-impact cardiovascular exercise, but the forward-leaning posture required by most racing-style bikes means that your head protrudes forward and isn't balanced on top of your neck as it should be. Neck strain is a likely result. Choose a bicycle with an upright handlebar position. Another option is a recumbent bicycle, which allows you to sit in a slightly reclined position with back support and your legs extended forward to pedal.

Neck injuries are most likely with sports that may lead to falls, such as skiing, and contact sports such as football, basketball, hockey, soccer, and lacrosse. Some activities that are notorious for straining the lower back, such as running and rowing, usually aren't particularly hard on the neck as long as you strive to keep your neck in a balanced, neutral position. Table 1, page 31, compares how common leisure activities affect your neck and provides pointers for neck-friendly participation. For all sports, proper conditioning to strengthen and stretch the neck muscles can help protect the neck.

If your neck is injured from playing sports, brisk walking is a good way to maintain your fitness level while your neck heals. Walking allows you to keep your head balanced at the top of your spine and doesn't require the impact of running or the twisting or turning of racquet sports or swimming.

Good nights for your neck

When it comes to easing neck pain, it's not only what you do during the day that counts, but also how you sleep at night.

Two sleeping positions are easiest on the neck: on your side or on your back. Whichever you prefer, choose an appropriate pillow. If you sleep on your back, choose a rounded pillow to support the natural curve of your neck, with a flatter pillow cushioning your head. This can be achieved by tucking a small neck roll into the pillowcase

Table 1: Neck health and common sports, exercise, and leisure activities

A number of common sports or activities can produce neck strain. Following are some tips to help you avoid problems.

ACTIVITY	NECK IMPACT	TIPS
Bicycling	When leaning over your handlebars in racing position, you might overly extend and strain your neck while trying to see the road. Rough terrain can be jarring.	• Change position frequently; avoid racing position and dropped handlebars. • Position your helmet for easy vision. • When experiencing neck problems, exercise on a recumbent bike or switch to an exercise bicycle and sit upright with your head balanced over your spine.
Gardening	Leaning forward for long periods can strain the neck, as can twisting and flexing the neck as you pull weeds.	• Use tools that allow you to stand upright. • Sit on a stool, or use positions such as kneeling or squatting instead of stooping over, to keep your neck in a neutral position. • Weed or dig when the ground is moist and soft.
Golf	Amateur golfers are less likely to strain their neck than their lower back. Turning your neck far to the side while it is flexed forward (in the backswing) can strain the neck.	• Minimize the time you let your neck hang; stand back slightly to address the ball with your neck in a more neutral position. • Shorten your backswing.
Swimming	Because water supports your back, swimming can be soothing, but each stroke has the potential to stress neck muscles. In the crawl, you may over-rotate the neck. In the breaststroke, the neck is extended. In the backstroke, you may strain to keep your head mostly out of the water.	• When doing the crawl, alternate breaths on the right and left sides, and turn your full body (not just your neck); alternatively, breathe through a snorkel and keep your neck in a neutral position. • When doing the backstroke, relax your neck and let the water support your head. • Avoid the breaststroke if you have neck pain, or learn to use your arms and chest muscles to lessen neck extension. • When your neck hurts, try water exercises that keep you upright.
Walking and running	If you tense your shoulders or thrust your head forward, you can strain your neck muscles.	• Keep your head upright and balanced over your spine with shoulders relaxed. Train your sights 10 to 20 feet ahead of you. • Consider single-vision glasses if bifocals make it necessary to bend your head to see the ground ahead. • Avoid hard running surfaces to minimize jarring. • When in pain, walk rather than run.
Yoga	Yoga can be an excellent way to loosen tight neck muscles and increase your range of motion. But forcing the neck into extreme positions can strain tight muscles and ligaments and put pressure on cervical discs.	• Work with a knowledgeable teacher to keep your shoulders down and your neck relaxed in various poses. Don't do any pose that causes pain. • Avoid positions that require substantial neck flexion (such as shoulder stand) or extension (such as backbends). Avoid headstands until you have sufficient arm and shoulder strength to take some of the weight off your head.

of a flatter, softer pillow, or by using a special pillow that has a built-in neck support with an indentation for the head to rest in. Feather pillows tend to easily conform to the shape of the neck. They will collapse over time, however, and should be replaced every year or so.

If you're looking for alternatives, another option is a traditionally shaped pillow with "memory foam" that conforms to the contour of your head and neck. Some cervical pillows are also made with memory foam. Manufacturers of memory foam pillows claim they help foster proper spinal alignment. Avoid using too high or stiff a pillow, which keeps the neck flexed overnight and can result in morning pain and stiffness.

If you sleep on your side, keep your spine straight by using a pillow that is higher under your neck than your head. Sleeping on your stomach is tough on your spine, because the back is arched and your neck turned to the side. Preferred sleeping positions are often set early in life and can be tough to change, not to mention that we don't often wake up in the same position in which we fell asleep. Still, it's worth trying to start the night sleeping on your back or side in a well-supported, healthy position.

When you are riding in a plane, train, or car, or even just reclining to watch TV, a horseshoe-shaped pillow can support your neck and prevent your head from dropping to one side if you doze. If the pillow is too large behind the neck, however, it will force your head forward.

Emerging research suggests that not just sleep position, but also sleep quality, can play a role in musculoskeletal pain, including neck pain. In one study, researchers compared musculoskeletal pain in 4,140 healthy men and women with and without sleeping problems. Sleeping problems included difficulty falling asleep, trouble staying asleep, waking early in the mornings, and nonrestorative sleep. The researchers found that people who reported moderate to severe problems in at least three of these four categories were significantly more likely to develop chronic musculoskeletal pain after one year than those who reported little or no trouble with sleep. One possible explanation is that sleep disturbances disrupt the muscle relaxation and healing that normally occur during sleep. Additionally, it is well established that pain can disrupt sleep, contributing to a vicious circle of pain disrupting sleep and sleep problems contributing to pain.

Pain medications

Medication, in combination with a program of exercise and ergonomic improvements, can be an effective solution to chronic or recurring neck pain. There are many choices of medication, including some that aren't known primarily as pain relievers. But medications must be used with caution as they all carry risks. When recommending a specific drug, your doctor will want you to take the smallest dose required for the shortest amount of time necessary to relieve your pain.

Your clinician bases a recommendation for medication on whether your pain is longstanding or started recently, whether it stems from your joints and soft tissues or from your nerves or spinal cord, and whether you have other symptoms or diseases that might be more compatible with a particular drug. Medication choice can involve a certain amount of trial and error. If you try one medication and it doesn't relieve your symptoms or it causes unacceptable side effects, don't wait for your next appointment to ask for help; there are many choices and few rigid rules about which type works best for each individual. Over-the-counter pain relievers, used according to package directions, are effective for most kinds of neck pain. But if neck pain is related to an underlying disease, such as rheumatoid arthritis, you need to treat the disorder rather than just the pain.

A number of pain medications can cause physical dependence, a condition in which stopping abruptly will cause unpleasant withdrawal symptoms. But dependence is not the same as addiction. People who build up dependence can taper off the drug gradually under a doctor's supervision to avoid the side effects of abrupt withdrawal.

Acetaminophen

Acetaminophen (Tylenol) is usually the first choice for relief of neck pain because it is quite effective and doesn't cause the gastrointestinal bleeding and other side effects of aspirin and other NSAID pain relievers. It's not entirely clear how acetaminophen relieves pain. One possibility is that it raises the threshold at which you perceive pain signals. Another is that it reduces the production of chemical messengers that produce those pain signals. Acetaminophen does not reduce inflammation, but many cases of neck pain do not involve inflammation, so this is not a problem. Acetaminophen is non-addictive. For severe pain, it can be combined with opiate painkillers or NSAIDs.

On the downside, acetaminophen is processed by the liver, so it is not a good choice if you have liver disease or regularly drink more than a glass or two of alcohol per day. Overdose can cause liver damage. Regardless of whether you already have liver problems, you should stay within the limits of 1,000 milligrams (mg) at a time and 3,000 mg daily to avoid life-threatening liver damage. The daily limit was recently lowered from 4,000 mg after widespread reports of accidental overdose of the medication. It is important to note that many different drugs—as many as 600 over-the-counter and prescription medications, including cold, allergy and sleep medications—contain acetaminophen.

Nonsteroidal anti-inflammatory drugs

Known as NSAIDs, drugs of this diverse and popular class relieve pain and inhibit inflammation, and they are not addictive. At the low doses available over the counter, NSAIDs such as aspirin, ibuprofen (Advil, Motrin), naproxen sodium (Aleve, Anaprox), and others relieve pain about as well as acetaminophen. These medications are also available in prescription strength.

Another type of NSAID, the COX-2 inhibitor, is not used as frequently because of potential cardiovascular side effects, particularly in individuals who have a history of heart problems or who are at risk for heart disease. Celecoxib (Celebrex) is the only COX-2 inhibitor currently on the market, and it is available only by prescription. If you have a history of heart disease or are at risk for it, you should use a COX-2 inhibitor only when there are no other alternatives, and even in that case, only on a short-term basis. For instance, if traditional NSAIDs such as ibuprofen or naproxen cause stomach irritation, your first choice should be acetaminophen. Another way to offset the problem of gastrointestinal side effects is to combine a smaller dose of the NSAID with acetaminophen or to take the NSAID with a proton-pump inhibitor such as omeprazole (Prilosec), which reduces the production of stomach acid.

Problems with COX-2 drugs have cast a shadow over older NSAIDs as well, raising concerns about their potential association with heart disease. In fact, several reports have identified a few of the traditional NSAIDs—including ibuprofen, naproxen, and diclofenac (Voltaren)—with an increased risk for heart disease. Yet other studies have vindicated naproxen, which may be the safest of the bunch. More long-term studies are needed to provide conclusive answers about the impact of traditional NSAIDs on the heart. In the meantime, it is imperative to discuss the risks of NSAIDs with your doctor, who can determine which pain reliever is appropriate for you.

Another medical risk associated with long-term use of NSAIDs is the possibility of kidney damage. If you have kidney disease or are over age 65, your doctor should test your blood regularly for signs of kidney damage and may suggest an alternative medication if you need long-term pain treatment.

If you take a daily low-dose aspirin to protect your heart, note that taking another NSAID (whether over-the-counter or prescribed by your doctor) at the same time can interfere with aspirin's blood-thinning benefits. You should wait at least 30 minutes after taking aspirin to take another NSAID. Alternatively, you can take aspirin eight hours after taking another NSAID.

Take NSAIDs as needed only for the duration of your neck pain. Talk to your doctor about how to schedule your NSAIDs: taking them on a regular schedule may be more helpful than waiting until the pain becomes intolerable. Remember that not all NSAIDs are the same. People respond to each one differently, so if one NSAID is ineffective for your neck pain or causes side effects, another may work better.

Topical anti-inflammatories

Note that there are also topical analgesics that contain salicylate (a form of the active ingredient in aspirin). These can help relieve neck pain associated with arthritis and may reduce joint inflammation. These creams, ointments, and salves, sold under such brand names as Bengay and Aspercreme, are rubbed directly into the skin at the site of discomfort. Talk to your doctor before using such medications if you are allergic to aspirin or are taking blood thinners.

While topical NSAID treatments containing the prescription drug diclofenac are also available, they are not commonly used for neck pain.

Muscle relaxants

Painful muscle spasms can be treated with any of several unrelated medications called muscle relaxants. These medications work on the brain to promote general relaxation. Some muscle relaxants can cause dependence; they usually are taken for only a short period of time soon after the onset of pain. Muscle relaxants typically are prescribed in conjunction with rest, physical therapy, and other measures to relieve pain and muscle spasm related to neck muscle injury.

Cyclobenzaprine (Flexeril) reduces neck pain and can also help with difficulty sleeping. This medication causes drowsiness and sometimes leads to urinary retention in men with large prostate glands. If you are age 65 or older, try to avoid this drug, as it as not as safe and effective as other medications. Elderly people may be more sensitive to serious side effects associated with the use of cyclobenzaprine, although a low dose (e.g., 5 mg/day) may be well tolerated. A related drug called carisoprodol (Soma) is usually prescribed for a limited period because it can be habit-forming. It should not be taken with other substances that can make you sleepy, such as alcohol, narcotics, benzodiazepines (often used as sleep medications and sedatives), and other muscle relaxants.

Diazepam (Valium) is a muscle relaxant in the benzodiazepine group sometimes prescribed for a short period to relieve neck pain with spasms. This medication is used with caution because it is habit-forming, can interfere with normal sleep patterns, and makes you drowsy.

Other muscle relaxants, developed for use in people with severe, painful muscle spasms related to multiple sclerosis or spinal cord injury, are sometimes prescribed for neck pain. These medications—baclofen (Lioresal) and tizanidine (Zanaflex)—work by binding to specific receptors in the brain and spinal cord, dampening nerve signals to the muscles. The side effects include drowsiness and confusion. These medications interact with alcohol and many other drugs, including sedatives, tricyclic antidepressants, and treatments for high blood pressure, Parkinson's disease, and bipolar disorder. Tizanidine should not be taken with the antidepressant fluvoxamine (Luvox) or the antibiotic ciprofloxacin (Cipro). Metaxalone (Skelaxin) is another option for relief of neck pain that is sometimes prescribed as an adjunct to rest, physical therapy, and other measures. Its mode of action hasn't been clearly identified, but may be related to its sedative properties. Side effects can include nausea, vomiting, gastrointestinal upset, drowsiness, dizziness, headache, and nervousness.

Opioids

The most powerful pain relievers—a large class of drugs called opioid medications—are available by prescription only. These drugs have morphine-like properties and are used only for severe pain. Opioids do not reduce inflammation. Rather, they work by interacting with the receptors on brain and spinal cord nerves for endogenous opioids—the body's natural painkilling substances. Some examples of opioid medications are codeine (Tylenol No. 3 and others), hydrocodone (Lortab, Vicodin), oxycodone (Oxycontin, Percocet, Percodan, Roxicodone), and hydromorphone (Dilaudid and others). A related medication, tramadol (Ultram), also acts on opioid receptors but is not considered an opioid.

Care must be taken with opioids to avoid dependence, which may develop in as little as two weeks. Therefore, opioids are usually reserved for short-term treatment of severe neck pain or after neck surgery. Long-term opioid therapy is occasionally used to treat chronic, intractable pain, but only in carefully selected and monitored individuals. Because of increasing concern about opioid dependence, your physician may be reluctant to prescribe this type of medication.

Because opioids may cause physical dependence, you can develop withdrawal symptoms if you stop using them suddenly. For your safety, your doctor will suggest tapering off slowly if you have used the drugs for several weeks or at high doses.

In addition to dependence, there are other problems with these drugs. Side effects such as dizziness and drowsiness can make it difficult for people to participate in physical therapy while taking these medications; nausea and constipation are also common adverse effects. Older individuals are particularly sensitive to opioids and require lower doses. Many opioid preparations include acetaminophen, so additional acetaminophen should be avoided.

Antidepressants and anticonvulsants

Aside from their primary actions, some antidepressant and anticonvulsant medications help relieve pain.

Tricyclic antidepressants, such as amitriptyline (Elavil and others), desipramine (Norpramin), and nortriptyline (Pamelor), increase pain tolerance. The tricyclic antidepressants relieve nerve pain at a dose one-half to one-third of the dose needed to treat depression. They also work faster for pain than for depression. The major side effect is drowsiness, which can be useful for people who have trouble sleeping because of chronic pain. Other side effects include dry mouth and weight gain.

Although not specifically approved for neck pain, selective serotonin reuptake inhibitors (SSRIs) such as fluoxetine (Prozac) are sometimes prescribed for chronic pain. It's not clear exactly how they help manage pain, but they appear to affect transmission of pain signals to the brain.

Two serotonin-norepinephrine reuptake inhibitors (SNRIs), duloxetine (Cymbalta) and milnacip-

Table 2: Drugs used to treat neck pain

This table provides examples of drugs in each category and is not intended to be a comprehensive list.

GENERIC NAME (BRAND NAME)	USES	SIDE EFFECTS
Analgesic		
acetaminophen (Tylenol and many brands of pain relievers, cold medicines, and sleep remedies)	Relieves pain caused by injury, osteoarthritis, or other conditions.	Can be used in conjunction with NSAIDs. Less likely to cause gastric bleeding than other pain relievers, but may cause nausea, vomiting, diarrhea, jaundice, rash, tiredness, weakness. Excess dosages can cause liver damage. Heavy drinkers should be particularly careful about taking acetaminophen.
Nonsteroidal anti-inflammatory drugs (NSAIDs)		
aspirin (many brand names) **ibuprofen** (Advil, Motrin, Nuprin) **indomethacin** (Indocin) **naproxen** (Aleve, Anaprox, others)	Reduce inflammation and relieve pain by inhibiting prostaglandins, which are involved in the body's inflammatory response.	Stomach pain, gastric bleeding, nausea, drowsiness, dizziness, fluid retention, diarrhea, constipation, blurred vision. High doses can cause ringing in the ears. People who are allergic to aspirin, have kidney disease, or take blood thinners should not take NSAIDs. People who take NSAIDs regularly should be monitored for gastric bleeding and liver or kidney damage. Some NSAIDs may also cause an increased risk of cardiovascular disease.
Selective NSAID (COX-2 inhibitor)		
celecoxib (Celebrex)	Reduces inflammation and relieves pain by inhibiting prostaglandins, which are involved in the body's inflammatory response.	Side effects are similar to NSAIDs (above) but with fewer severe gastrointestinal problems. People allergic to sulfa drugs should not take celecoxib. May have cardiovascular side effects. Discuss your health risks with your doctor before using.
Muscle relaxants		
carisoprodol (Soma, others) **cyclobenzaprine** (Flexeril) **diazepam** (Valium, others) **metaxalone** (Skelaxin) **methocarbamol** (Robaxin)	Relax muscles and ease pain associated with muscle strains, spasms, and injuries.	Dizziness, drowsiness, stomach upset, heartburn, constipation, headache. Metaxalone can cause headache and nervousness or irritability. Cyclobenzaprine can cause urinary retention in men with large prostates. Diazepam is a depressant and can be habit-forming.
baclofen (Lioresal) **tizanidine** (Zanaflex)	Relax muscles and ease pain associated with muscle strains, spasms, and injuries.	Drowsiness and confusion. Tell your doctor if you are taking medicine for hypertension, Parkinson's disease, or bipolar illness or if you use alcohol, sedatives, or antidepressants.
Antidepressants		
Tricyclic antidepressants		
amitriptyline (Elavil, others) **desipramine** (Norpramin) **imipramine** (Tofranil) **nortriptyline** (Aventyl, Pamelor)	At low doses, may increase pain tolerance.	Drowsiness, anxiety, restlessness, dry mouth, constipation, urinary retention, weight gain.
Selective serotonin reuptake inhibitors (SSRIs)		
citalopram (Celexa) **fluoxetine** (Prozac) **paroxetine** (Paxil) **sertraline** (Zoloft)	May provide pain relief independent of effects on mood.	Nausea, loss of appetite, diarrhea, dry mouth, trouble sleeping, dizziness, drowsiness, yawning, weakness, sweating. Serious side effects can include unusual or severe behavior or mood changes, weight loss, change in sexual ability, vision changes. Rare but serious side effects include uncontrolled movements (e.g., tremor), fever or flu-like symptoms, muscle stiffness, fast or irregular heartbeats, chest pain, easy bruising or bleeding, unusual bleeding, and seizures.

continued on page 37

Table 2 *continued*

GENERIC NAME (BRAND NAME)	USES	SIDE EFFECTS
Serotonin-norepinephrine reuptake inhibitors (SNRIs)		
duloxetine (Cymbalta) **milnacipran** (Savella)	May provide pain relief independent of effects on mood.	Nausea, dry mouth, constipation, loss of appetite, fatigue, drowsiness, dizziness, increased sweating, blurred vision, rash, itching. Rare but serious side effects include stomach pain, yellowing of the eyes/skin, dark urine, seizures, fast heartbeat, mood changes, sleeplessness, irritability, angry feelings, restlessness, impulsive action, rapid speech.
Anticonvulsants		
gabapentin (Neurontin)	Relieves nerve-related pain, including cervical radiculopathy.	Drowsiness, tiredness, weakness, dizziness, headache, uncontrollable shaking, double or blurred vision, unsteadiness, anxiety, memory problems, strange thoughts, unwanted eye movements, nausea, vomiting, heartburn, diarrhea, dry mouth, constipation, weight gain, swelling, back or joint pain, fever, runny nose, ear pain, red or itchy eyes. Serious side effects include rash, itching, swelling of the face, hoarseness, difficulty swallowing or breathing, and seizures.
pregabalin (Lyrica)	Reduces pain and improves function in people with fibromyalgia, possibly by decreasing the number of pain signals sent out by nerves in the body; relieves nerve pain.	Tiredness, dizziness, headache, dry mouth, nausea, vomiting, constipation, gas, bloating, elevated mood, speech problems, confusion, anxiety, weakness. Serious side effects include blurred vision, hives, rash, blisters, shortness of breath, wheezing, and chest pain.
Opioids		
codeine (Tylenol No. 3, others) **hydrocodone** (Vicodin, Lortab) **hydromorphone** (Dilaudid) **oxycodone** (Oxycontin, Percocet, Percodan, Roxicet)	Provide stronger pain relief by interacting with opiate receptors in the brain; usually used only for brief periods.	Nausea, dizziness or lightheadedness, vomiting, euphoria, constipation, abdominal pain, rash, headache. Can be habit-forming when taken over time. Should be used cautiously by people with liver disease or a history of substance abuse. Can cause seizures. May interact with other medications and alcohol. Long-term use may cause more serious side effects.
tramadol (Ultram)	Non-opioid but acts on opioid receptors.	
Corticosteroids		
oral corticosteroids such as prednisone (Orasone, Prelone, Cortan, Deltasone, Liquid Pred)	Reduce inflammation.	If taken at low doses for a week or less, side effects are uncommon; therapy for several months or years may cause more serious side effects such as fluid retention, facial hair growth, easy bruising, osteoporosis, cataracts, acne, sleeplessness, muscle wasting, headache, and glucose intolerance. Should be reduced gradually if taken for more than 10 to 14 days. Long-term use may cause more serious side effects.
injectable corticosteroids	Relieve pain and suppress inflammation.	Tenderness, burning, or tingling at injection site. Risk of joint infections or cartilage damage when injected into joints, tendon sheaths, or bursae. The systemic side effects that appear with oral use seldom occur with occasional injectable use.

ran (Savella), are approved for the treatment of fibromyalgia, which is often associated with chronic neck pain, in addition to widespread pain throughout the body.

Anticonvulsant medications treat seizure disorders, but they are also used for several types of nerve-related pain, including cervical radiculopathy. Gabapentin is often the first anticonvulsant used for nerve pain because it has fewer side effects than other anticonvulsant medications. The anticonvulsant drug pregabalin (Lyrica) also has FDA approval for the treatment of fibromyalgia.

Corticosteroids

Corticosteroids, such as prednisone, reduce pain by lowering the body's ability to generate inflammation. When first introduced in the 1950s, corticosteroids were regarded as miracle drugs because of their dramatic effect on people with active rheumatoid arthritis. However, within a few years it became clear that long-term use of oral corticosteroids has serious side effects: bone weakening, compression fractures of the back, diabetes, increased susceptibility to infections, cataracts, hypertension, and other health problems.

Injections of corticosteroids into joints provide pain relief with fewer side effects than oral versions. For neck pain, injection into facet joints or the epidural space can quickly relieve pain in some situations (see "Injectable drugs," below). Although most side effects occur when these drugs are taken orally, repeated corticosteroid injections into a joint can result in thinning of the cartilage and weakening of the ligaments.

Injectable drugs

Injection therapies bypass the digestive system, delivering pain-relieving medicine directly to the muscle or joint or to the epidural space in the spine. They can be helpful in treating neck pain from facet joint irritation, trigger points, spinal stenosis, or disc herniation.

Facet joint injections. To relieve painful facet joints, doctors sometimes inject a combination of a local anesthetic (such as lidocaine) and an inflammation-reducing corticosteroid into the joint. For the injection, you are given a sedative and then lie down on an x-ray table. Guided by x-ray, the physician (usually a pain expert or other specialist) inserts a very small needle into the joint. He or she may inject a small amount of dye to confirm proper needle placement before the medication is delivered. One or more facet joints may be treated in a single session. The procedure can be uncomfortable, but a local anesthetic is provided to limit pain. In addition to providing pain relief, facet joint injections may be used to diagnose a facet joint as the source of neck pain. Rapid relief is confirmation that the pain originated from the treated joint.

Trigger-point injections. Trigger points are tender, irritable nodules in muscles that are painful to the touch, with pain spreading to other nearby areas. Some doctors endorse the use of periodic trigger-point injections, but at this point there is no firm proof of long-term benefit. Trigger-point injection usually consists of a local anesthetic such as lidocaine or bupivacaine. Some doctors simply insert needles or inject a saline solution, without using a drug at all, but a systematic review found lidocaine injections to work better than needle insertion without injection for short-term pain relief. Trigger-point injections can be performed in the doctor's office, and more than one point may be injected in a single visit. With the injection, you may briefly feel referred pain from the spot, as well as a transient burning sensation until the anesthetic takes effect. Afterward, your doctor instructs you how to use ice and gentle stretching of the area to maximize the benefits of the injection. Trigger-point injections carry a small risk of side effects, including infection, increased pain, bleeding, and thinning or discoloration of the skin around the injection site.

Epidural injections. When neck and arm pain result from stenosis of the cervical spine or a herniated disc, doctors sometimes inject medication into the epidural space, which lies between the vertebrae and the protective coating of the spinal cord. Injections into the epidural space do not come in direct contact with nerve cells of the spinal cord. Injections typically include both an anesthetic to relieve pain and a steroid to reduce inflammation.

Epidural injections require skill and training. If you are undergoing an epidural injection to treat pain, you lie on an x-ray table and may take a sedating medication. The anesthesiologist or other physician cleanses the area. Guided by fluoroscopy (an x-ray procedure for viewing structures in motion), the doctor inserts a needle through the neck or back into the epidural space, injecting the medication as close as possible to the damaged disc or inflamed nerve root. To reduce the risk of bleeding or injury to the spinal cord, you refrain from taking aspirin or related medications for at least a week before the procedure. During the procedure, you may feel pressure but usually not pain. Afterward, you should be able to move around and return home, although you may be asked to take it easy for a few days. The anesthetic provides some immediate relief, but the full benefit of the injection may not be apparent for three to seven days. If needed, the injection can be repeated once or twice, and the relief after subsequent injections may last longer.

Epidural steroid injections can sometimes relieve pain well enough to allow you to participate in needed physical therapy or to give a herniated disc time to heal. They may even provide enough relief to allow you to avoid surgery. The injections are not as effective in people who have already undergone disc surgery.

Selective nerve root blocks (transforaminal epidural injection). A selective nerve root block is a type of epidural injection that delivers a local anesthetic and steroid into an intervertebral foramen, the opening where a single nerve root exits the spine. The procedure must be performed by an experienced physician guided by x-ray fluoroscopy or CT scan. If a selective nerve root block immediately improves your symptoms, that helps confirm that a specific nerve root is causing them. This type of injection is often chosen when a disc has herniated into the intervertebral foramen. Some people are able to avoid surgery by undergoing a series of selective nerve blocks to give the herniated disc time to heal. It has also become an option for chronic neck pain caused by whiplash.

Complementary and alternative treatments

Pain is a complex response. On the most basic level, it conveys a simple message: "That flame is hot, take your hand away!" But many physiological and psychological factors can affect how keenly you feel a particular pain at a given time. Have you ever noticed that a throbbing pain seems to hurt more at night as you lie in bed than when you are up doing something interesting? This is an example of how your mind influences your perception of pain. What's more, sensitivity to pain varies from one person to the next, and some people are more adept at controlling their response to it.

That's where a variety of complementary and alternative treatments may help. They won't correct degenerative disc disease, for example. But they may help you relax tense muscles, relieve the anxiety associated with chronic pain, and gain a greater sense of well-being. According to a survey by the National Center for Health Statistics, back pain and neck pain are the top two reasons people visit complementary medicine providers.

The complementary and alternative therapies listed here are unlikely to cause harm, and many people find them helpful even though science has yet to determine their effectiveness. However, if you have certain neck conditions, you should be cautious about massage (see page 43). And you should avoid chiropractic manipulation if you have significant neck arthritis or any nerve involvement such as a pinched nerve, tingling, or shooting pain in the arm or leg (see "Caution on chiropractic," page 44).

Mind-body therapies

While a sudden stab of pain can be a good thing, alerting you that something is wrong, chronic pain may serve no important function, and it may continue long after an initial injury heals. No matter what started your pain, once pain becomes chronic, it can start a cascade of anxiety, depression, social isolation, and declining fitness—all of which may contribute to even more pain. The mind and body are part of an intimate, two-way network of influence and communication. Pain can cause a decline in emotional health, and emotional stress can contribute to and intensify chronic pain.

Because the mind and body are so closely interconnected, your doctor may recommend a combination of therapies that aim to soothe both the body and the soul.

Cognitive behavioral therapy

Cognitive behavioral therapy (CBT) is a widely accepted approach to gaining control over chronic pain. Based on the idea that your thoughts can influence your mood, how you experience pain, and how

When sympathy hurts

In cognitive behavioral therapy, you learn to be aware of how your thoughts and habits can either contribute to your pain or help ease it. In addition, the attitudes and responses of important people in your life can have a huge impact. Someone who loves you may inadvertently discourage you from gaining control over your pain if he or she promotes an endless quest for a medical fix, or offers help and understanding to the point of fostering dependence. Likewise, in the pursuit of a successful lawsuit, a lawyer may encourage you to perceive your neck problems as permanent and debilitating. This perception can interfere with your chances for managing your pain, gradually taking on more activities, and regaining a normal life. Generally speaking, if you stick to your routine as best you can—trying to work, continue with exercise, and keep your mind off of your condition—you will tend to improve more than those who allow the pain to get in the way of their day-to-day lives.

To gain maximum support, your physician or cognitive behavioral therapist may include key people in educational sessions about chronic pain and elicit their cooperation in achieving your goals.

fully you can function and cope with a chronic pain condition, CBT helps break negative patterns of thought and pain. For example, if your mind leaps to the worst-case scenario whenever neck pain recurs—"It will never get better," "I'll never go back to work"—that thought itself can intensify your pain experience and contribute to anxiety and depression. It can also pose a barrier to staying engaged with your work and social life and discourage you from taking action that might improve the pain, such as exercise.

In CBT, you spend several individual or group sessions (about an hour long) with a therapist. You may also have homework assignments between sessions. Through discussion, skills training, and homework, CBT teaches you to notice negative thoughts and reframe them in a more positive light—for example, "I am making progress to help myself feel better" or "Many people are able to get their neck pain under control and go back to work"—to help you manage your pain and participate as fully as possible in the activities you care about. In a 2015 Cochrane review of 10 studies, CBT was better than other interventions (such as medication, physical therapy, and exercise) at reducing fear of movement in people with chronic neck pain. While CBT was better than no treatment at reducing pain, replacing or adding CBT to other modes of treatment provided no added benefit.

Biofeedback

Biofeedback helps you gain conscious control over body processes that are normally unconscious, such as regulating blood pressure and the electrical activity in your muscles. Biofeedback can be useful in neck pain because it helps you learn to relax muscles that are constantly tight and strengthen those you don't use properly or have much awareness of. Though many people report benefit from biofeedback, there are not enough clinical data to support or refute the effectiveness of the therapy for the treatment of neck pain.

The biofeedback practitioner pastes electronic sensors on the skin over the muscles you commonly tense, such as the trapezius, and the electrical activity is translated into a visual signal or sound—the feedback—that lets you know the state of tension or relaxation in those muscles. The practitioner instructs you in relaxation techniques to reduce muscle tension, and as you apply them, you receive feedback from the machine on how much (or how little) the muscle is relaxing. Relaxing a habitually tense muscle in the neck may initially feel uncomfortable, but with the feedback, you know whether you're on the right track. To find a certified biofeedback practitioner, contact the Biofeedback Certification International Alliance (see "Resources," page 50).

Breathing exercises

Conscious, controlled breathing is a component of most relaxation techniques. Stress and anxiety are associated with rather quick and shallow "chest breathing," and this is the everyday breathing pattern for many people. By taking time to focus on breathing more deeply and slowly, from the diaphragm, you can elicit a nervous system response that helps reduce blood pressure and heart rate and encourages tense muscles to relax—particularly those of the neck, shoulders, and upper back. Deep breathing can be done in any position but may be easiest to start while lying on your back. Follow these steps:

- Breathe slowly in and out through your nostrils, keeping your inhale and exhale roughly the same length.
- Become aware of your breathing. Put your hand just below your navel and feel your abdomen gently rise and fall as you inhale and exhale.
- Inhale and exhale slowly and completely.

Qigong and yoga

Mindful movement practices are exercises performed precisely and with focused awareness. Often arising out of spiritual traditions, the practices can have physical benefits such as enabling you to relax and helping you train your body to move optimally during exercise and everyday activities.

Qigong is a therapeutic Chinese practice that involves slow movements, breathing exercises, and meditation. Tai chi is a well-known form of qigong. One small randomized controlled trial published in the journal *Spine* compared qigong with exercise therapy for the treatment of chronic neck pain. Participants were assigned to a maximum of 12 treatment sessions over three months with either qigong therapy or supervised exercise therapy. At six and 12 months after treatment, those in both the qigong and exercise therapy groups continued to have significant improvements compared with the beginning of the study. Improvements were seen in the following areas: average neck pain during the most recent week, current neck pain, average daily neck pain as noted in a neck pain diary, neck disability, and range of motion in neck rotation.

Yoga is an ancient practice combining exercises, breathing techniques, and meditation. Originating in India, it is currently practiced in many variations throughout the world. Iyengar yoga, a type that emphasizes very precise positioning, using props as needed to maintain proper alignment in yoga poses, is often recommended for people with painful conditions, such as fibromyalgia, lower back pain, and arthritis. In a recent randomized controlled trial involving people with chronic neck pain, participants who attended nine weeks of Iyengar yoga classes achieved less pain and better functioning than those in the control group, who received a self-care manual with home-based exercises. One year later, after everyone had been given the Iyengar yoga classes, participants maintained a significant reduction in pain intensity, with almost half reporting better than 50% improvement. Those who maintained a regular yoga practice after the nine weeks of classes gained the most benefit.

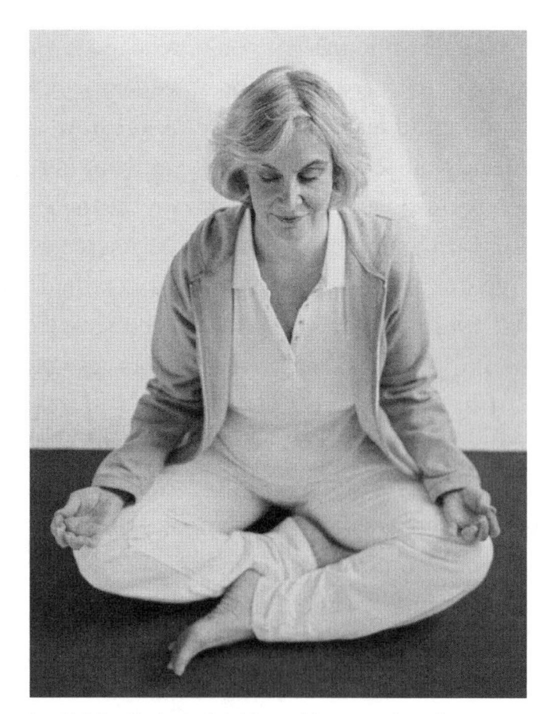

In addition to beneficial breathing practices, Iyengar yoga stresses posture and alignment, which may help people with neck pain.

Other therapies

Throughout history, people have developed a variety of methods for pain relief. It is not always clear why some of them work for some people at least some of the time. If you're interested in alternative treatments for neck problems and other painful conditions, the Arthritis Foundation (see "Resources," page 50) has published a guide on this topic and is a good source for balanced information on dietary supplements and other alternative therapies. Here are a few options.

Acupuncture

This ancient Chinese technique uses slim needles to stimulate precise points along the body's "energy meridians." According to practitioners, this corrects energy blockages and disease-causing imbalances. While you lie on a table, the acupuncturist inserts dozens of single-use, disposable needles along various meridians all over the body and typically leaves them in place for 20 to 30 minutes. Often a low-level current is also applied to the needles, which may produce a slight tingling sensation. Some scientific studies confirm that acupuncture can play a role in pain relief, possibly by releasing endorphins, natural morphine-like chemicals in the nervous system.

A National Institutes of Health consensus panel concluded that acupuncture is a reasonable alternative or adjunct treatment for many kinds of pain, including low back pain and pain stemming from osteoarthritis and fibromyalgia. Research specifically on neck pain is limited. However, a study that examined 14 clinical trials found acupuncture to be effective against chronic pain in the neck. Together, the trials included 4,249 participants who received acupuncture for neck pain that had lasted for one month or more. People who received acupuncture reported better pain relief immediately after treatment and in the short term than those who received massage, traction, or sham treatments—such as acupuncture needles inserted in the wrong places, sham laser, or sham TENS. The study documented no significant improvement in long-term pain relief or disability. In a 2015 longer-term study, however, people with neck pain lasting at least three months (half of participants had been in pain for six years or more) gained relief from up to 12 acupuncture sessions in addition to usual care (such as prescription medication and physical therapy). What's more, they continued to have less pain and disability at one year than those who received only standard treatments. Results were on a par with those of participants who received training in the Alexander Technique (see below).

If you want to try acupuncture, choose a licensed acupuncturist, or, if your state does not require a license, choose one that is certified by the National Certification Commission for Acupuncture and Oriental Medicine (see "Resources," page 50). Insurers often cover acupuncture for specific conditions, including fibromyalgia and myofascial pain.

Alexander Technique

In a series of one-on-one sessions, Alexander Technique instructors use hands-on cues and verbal instructions to teach people how to avoid unnecessary muscle tension and to improve posture and body alignment when engaging in everyday activities—whether sitting at the computer or playing a musical instrument that can place special stress on the neck. The technique was developed decades ago by an actor who experienced recurrent hoarseness and who traced the problem to the way he constricted the muscles in his throat when he projected his voice. He found that he could eliminate the problem by improving his posture and using his muscles differently.

In the 2015 study of acupuncture described above, one group of participants attended up to 20 Alexander Technique lessons in addition to receiving their usual care. After one year, their reductions in neck pain and disability were similar to those of participants who underwent acupuncture—and were significantly better than those seen in people who received only standard care.

Not all trials have shown a benefit, however. In a 2016 study comparing five Alexander Technique lessons to an equal amount of time applying heat to painful areas, participants receiving both treatments had improvement in their chronic neck pain, with a reduction of about 20% on a pain intensity scale. However, the Alexander technique students ranked significantly higher on measures of their physical quality of life.

If you want to try the Alexander Technique, look for a certified teacher who has completed a three-year training course. A teacher locator is available on the website of the American Society for the Alexander Technique (see "Resources," page 50). Be aware, however, that insurers do not usually cover Alexander Technique lessons, citing inadequate evidence of their effectiveness in the peer-reviewed medical literature.

Massage

In massage therapy, a massage therapist applies hands-on pressure to the skin and soft tissues. Massage may help promote general well-being and healing by relieving muscle tension and spasm, loosening stiff joints, and promoting relaxation. It is one of the most popular alternative therapies for both neck and back pain, which account for about one-third of more than 100 million annual visits to massage therapists in the United States.

Despite its popularity, there are not many high-quality studies focusing on the value of massage in treating neck pain. There are a few small trials, however. One 2014 study of 228 adults with neck pain persisting for at least three months found that therapeutic massage was safe and beneficial in treating chronic neck pain in the short term—but it took a lot of massage to ease the pain. The study divided participants into six groups. Five of the groups received four weeks of treatment involving various amounts of massage (30-minute massages two to three times a week, or 60-minute massages once, twice, or three times a week). The final group was placed on a waiting list. Compared with the wait-list group, only those who had received 60-minute treatments two or three times a week experienced a significant improvement in pain intensity or neck function one week after the course of treatment had ended. In a 2015 follow-up study that provided six weekly 60-minute "booster" massage treatments to participants in all groups, only those initially assigned to one of the 60-minute massage groups benefited from the booster treatments.

While massage is safe for most people, it should not be done directly over a tumor, recent incision, open wound, or swollen or bruised tissues. And anyone with neck pain who opts for massage therapy should keep in mind that the structures of the neck encompass a tighter space than in the back, making them more prone to injury. For this reason, you should use caution with massage, especially deep tissue massage, and tell the therapist right away if you experience any pain during the treatment. If you have been diagnosed with neck arthritis, check with your doctor before having massage therapy on your neck. The American Massage Therapy Association (see "Resources," page 50) can help you find a massage therapist who graduated from a certified program and is licensed in your state or locality, if licensing is required by local law.

Caution on chiropractic

Avoid chiropractic manipulation if you have osteoporosis or rheumatoid arthritis, or if there is a chance that your neck pain stems from significant arthritis, infection, or fracture. If you have neurological symptoms along with neck pain—such as tingling or numbness—you should not undergo chiropractic manipulation. Very rarely, chiropractic manipulations can worsen or even cause disc herniation, nerve root irritation, or spinal cord injury. Among the most serious and rare complications of chiropractic manipulation of the neck is vertebral or carotid artery dissection, a tearing of one of the two major arteries supplying blood to the brain, which can lead to stroke. Neurological symptoms of this life-threatening condition may occur immediately or up to a week or more after the adjustment. Experts advise that chiropractors avoid one particular movement, called rotational thrust, on the neck, and use no manipulation of the neck on people with serious degenerative disease.

Chiropractic manipulation

In a 2015 national Gallup survey, about half of adults report having been treated by a chiropractor at some point in their lives, and 29% say a chiropractor would be their first choice of a health provider if they experienced back or neck pain. Chiropractic therapy aims to relieve symptoms and encourage normal spine function for many types of neck pain, primarily through manipulation of the spine (called adjustment).

The particular technique used for manipulation varies based on a number of factors, including a person's underlying condition and other anatomical considerations. In several techniques used on the cervical spine, a chiropractor uses his or her hands or a mechanical device to deliver a quick thrust to slightly move the vertebrae neighboring a restricted joint. Greater force may be used in certain situations, for example, to correct misalignment of a cervical vertebra.

Another technique known as the Cox technique does not involve high-velocity thrusting. Rather, it combines gentle pressure with subtle flexing and stretching maneuvers. Chiropractors sometimes use the Cox technique for disc injuries, facet joint pain, and whiplash injuries.

Despite its popularity, some medical experts advise against high-velocity chiropractic manipulation for neck pain, especially in people with neck arthritis, because of rare but potentially serious complications (see "Caution on chiropractic," above). For this reason, have a medical evaluation of your neck pain before seeking chiropractic care, especially if you have symptoms that could indicate a condition for which chiropractic care might be particularly hazardous (see "When to seek immediate medical attention," page 6).

Many people gain relief from chiropractic care. However, well-controlled studies do not demonstrate greater value of chiropractic manipulation over other techniques (such as exercise therapy or physical therapy) in easing neck pain. For example, in a yearlong study that enrolled people with neck pain that had persisted for several weeks, chiropractic adjustments helped more than medication, but were no more effective than home exercise instructions. Even when compared with gentle neck mobilization (as might be done by a physical therapist), chiropractic manipulation was not found to be any better.

Chiropractors are state-licensed. Insurance coverage for chiropractic services is often available.

Dietary supplements

Many dietary supplements are promoted for their ability to reduce the pain and inflammation of arthritis; some people turn to them in an attempt to relieve neck pain. Many of these products lack good scientific support for neck pain relief. Some are harmless, but others can have side effects or interact with other medications, so it is important to talk with your doctor about any supplements you may be taking, particularly if you take any prescription or over-the-counter medications. An important factor to consider when choosing these remedies is that no governmental body controls the quality or amount of active ingredients in them. If you are a buyer, be aware that tests by independent laboratories have reported that the strengths listed on the label frequently do not match the amount in the bottle.

Glucosamine and chondroitin sulfate. Glucosamine and chondroitin sulfate are popular supplements used to address pain and loss of function from osteoarthritis. Glucosamine is a substance normally found in both cartilage and the lubricating fluid inside joints. Chondroitin sulfate is one component of a protein that makes cartilage elastic. It isn't clear how supplements of these nutrients might work, but it's possible that they encourage cartilage formation and minimize further breakdown while also reducing inflammation. Glucosamine and chondroitin sulfate are often used for arthritis in the hips and knees, and there is some evidence that glucosamine can reduce pain; however, claims that these supplements heal damaged joints or prevent future joint degeneration remain unproven. There are no high-quality studies of glucosamine or chondroitin as a treatment for neck pain.

Common side effects include intestinal gas and softened stools. Chondroitin sulfate structurally resembles the anticlotting drug heparin; if you're taking blood-thinning medication, check with your doctor before taking chondroitin. Because glucosamine can worsen diabetes, watch blood sugar levels carefully. Glucosamine is manufactured from shellfish, so people with shellfish allergies can react to it. In addition, studies show that the amount of glucosamine present in the products available in stores varies widely among manufacturers and possibly from batch to batch within the same brand, so it's difficult to know how much you're getting when you use this product.

Surgery for neck pain

Many people have neck pain, but only a small fraction of them require—or can even benefit from—surgery. Increasingly, doctors emphasize nonsurgical treatments for neck pain and, except in cases of severe injury, you can take the time to give them a try before considering surgery.

For example, if your symptoms result from a pinched nerve, you may be a candidate for surgery only after medications, physical therapy, and other treatments have failed. Mild myelopathy can also improve with closely monitored nonsurgical treatment. If you have significant pain or neurological symptoms that can be clearly linked to a correctable problem seen on imaging studies, surgery may be an option. Surgeons consider surgery earlier in individuals with compression of the spinal cord in order to avoid the possibility of permanent nerve damage.

If your neck pain is caused by degenerative disc disease, the benefits of surgery are uncertain, and doctors recommend a long and thorough trial of nonsurgical approaches first, resorting to an operation only if your pain is severe and unrelenting despite treatment.

Both neurosurgeons and orthopedic surgeons operate on the neck; some complete a fellowship program to specialize in spine surgery. If you do require surgery, you and your surgeon face many choices and evolving techniques.

Types of surgery

For some surgical procedures, the surgeon can cut through either the back or front of your neck to make repairs on the spine. Operating from the front, the surgeon must avoid injuring the windpipe and esophagus, but this approach is usually preferred because there is minimal damage to muscles and a low risk of significant blood loss. Many types of spinal surgery can be performed from the front, and the discs are more visible, but fusing the vertebrae is often necessary afterward to prevent instability. Operating from the back, the surgeon may be able to repair a herniated disc or remove bone spurs or tissues impinging on nerves without requiring fusion, thus speeding recovery and leaving the neck more flexible.

For some procedures, a full incision is no longer necessary. For example, portions of a damaged or bulging disc can be removed through a mini-incision rather than an open procedure, allowing quicker recovery and avoiding the need for hospital admission. Another option is laser spine surgery, which uses a focused beam of light to cut away soft tissues. But although it is heavily advertised, it has not been critically compared with non-laser surgery for neck pain, and it has limitations. For example, the devices cannot cut through bone and do not eliminate the need for an incision.

Because of the many options in spinal surgery, seek the opinion of more than one specialist. Following are short descriptions of some of the most common surgical procedures for neck pain.

Anterior discectomy. When a disc is pressing on one or more nerve roots, resulting in pain and significant neurological symptoms, a surgeon may remove the disc, a procedure called discectomy (see Figure 6, page 47). While you are under general anesthesia, the surgeon makes an incision in the front of your neck and separates the tissues to reach the front of the spine. The disc and any bone spurs impinging on the nerve or spinal cord are removed. Afterward, the space between the vertebrae is refilled to stabilize the area (see "Cervical spinal fusion," page 47). When the surgeon enters the neck from the front, there is a small possibility of injury to the esophagus or of short- or long-term hoarseness from injury to the nerves supplying the vocal cords.

Laminectomy. Laminectomy is a procedure to gain access to the discs and spinal cord from the back. The surgeon cuts vertically through the bony plates

Figure 6: Discectomy

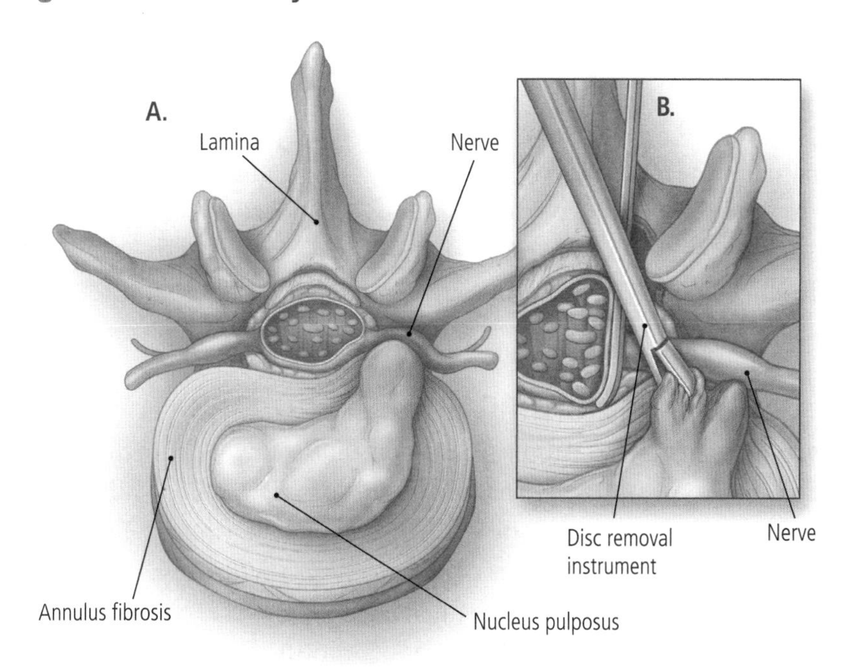

A. When a disc is herniated, the material within the disk (nucleus pulposus) bulges into the opening between vertebrae through which nerves leave the spine and extend to other parts of the body. This presses on the nerve root, causing pain.

B. During a discectomy, a portion of the bony arch of the vertebra (lamina) is removed, a procedure known as a laminectomy. This allows the surgeon to reach and remove the disc material causing the nerve-root compression.

(laminae) of the vertebra on both sides, removing the center section along with the bony projections toward the back of the vertebra (the parts you can feel when you run your fingers along the back of your spine). This creates an opening that relieves pressure on the spinal cord, and allows access for the surgeon to cut away all or part of a damaged disc and any bone spurs that are pressing on the spinal nerve roots. If the laminectomy involves several vertebrae, it can leave the spine unstable. To prevent this, the surgeon may perform a cervical spinal fusion (see below right).

Posterior keyhole foraminotomy. In some cases, depending on the direction in which the disc protrudes, a minimally invasive procedure called posterior keyhole foraminotomy is recommended. This procedure is a less risky alternative to anterior discectomy and laminectomy, but it is only an option when the disc bulges to the left or the right; repairing a central herniation (when the disc protrudes in the center) is more complicated and generally requires open surgery. While you are under general anesthesia, the surgeon, using x-ray guidance, makes a small, 2-centimeter incision on the back of your neck and inserts a tube down along the back of the spine. Through this tube, part of the bone and spurs as well as any protruding part of the disc are removed from the compressed nerves. Then the tube is removed and the incision is closed. No cervical spinal fusion is necessary.

Laminoplasty. Laminoplasty is surgery to create more room for the spinal cord. Laminoplasty is an option for people with severe spinal stenosis that is compressing the spinal cord and creating severe or progressive symptoms, such as pain, weakness in the arms or legs, and an unsteady gait. In this procedure, the surgeon relieves compression of the spine and then stabilizes the area. The surgeon cuts the tips off the bony processes at the back of each affected vertebra, notches the bony plate (lamina) of the vertebra on one side to create a hinge, and cuts the lamina all the way through on the other side, opening up the middle section like a door to relieve pressure on the spinal cord. Wedges of bone are inserted so that the channel for the spinal cord remains larger when the "door" is closed again.

Cervical spinal fusion. Fusion, also called arthrodesis, is a surgical procedure to join together selected vertebrae. Surgeons may perform this procedure if your neck is unstable as a result of fracture, if you have a disease such as rheumatoid arthritis, or if you are having surgery to relieve pressure on the spinal cord or remove a damaged disc.

To perform fusion, the surgeon connects neighboring vertebrae with metal implants or bone grafts (taken from the hip or elsewhere in the body or obtained from a bone bank). To prevent slippage during the healing process, a small metal plate is attached with screws. After surgery, the patient remains in the hospital for a short stay and wears a collar to hold the neck steady during recovery.

One technique may help certain people eliminate some of the risks involved with bone grafts (such as surgery at a second site on the body or rejection of a donor graft). During spinal fusion surgery, surgeons place bone proteins, often encased in collagen putty or sponges, in the affected areas of the spine. These proteins are called bone morphogenic proteins because they stimulate bone generation, making bone grafts unnecessary. Results from a small study found cervical spinal fusion performed with bone morphogenic proteins to be as effective as fusion performed with a bone graft from a person's own body.

Fusion limits flexibility in the neck, but usually this does not significantly interfere with activities. Because fusion places added stress on the joints above and below those that were fused, some patients develop deterioration of the nearby vertebrae over time and require another operation.

Laser-assisted disc decompression. This outpatient procedure, also known as intradiscal electrothermal therapy, is an older and less effective therapy that is still sometimes used. The surgeon uses a laser to vaporize a portion of the nucleus pulposus, the squishy interior of an intervertebral disc. The procedure is intended to ease the pain of a herniated disc by reducing internal pressure so the bulging edge recedes and no longer presses on nearby nerves. Your doctor may consider this procedure if you have a bulging disc that has not broken through the outer disc coating, if nonsurgical therapy has been unsuccessful, and if you have neurological symptoms that correspond to the location of the herniated disc. The procedure is less likely to help if the disc herniation is large, if there are other degenerative changes, or if more than one disc is involved.

To perform laser-assisted disc decompression, the doctor makes a small incision in the back, then puts a hollow needle into the disc and inserts a fiber-optic cable through it so the laser energy can be applied to vaporize the disc nucleus. This means of reaching the disc is called a percutaneous approach. This short outpatient procedure can be performed under local anesthesia, and recovery takes only a few days. Alternatively, percutaneous disc decompression may be performed using traditional surgical tools rather than a laser. Results are comparable.

Emerging surgical options

Medical specialists continue to invent new treatments and improve the options for treating neck pain.

Artificial discs. Some people who are faced with the prospect of having a spinal fusion have another alternative—artificial discs.

The FDA has approved the use of artificial discs for the surgical treatment of cervical degenerative disc disease. Clinical trials found that artificial disc replacement surgery improved neck pain, arm pain, or both, and that it was as safe and effective as standard surgery.

Traditionally, a discectomy is performed to remove a diseased or bulging disc that is putting pressure on nerve roots or the spinal cord. The neighboring vertebrae are then joined with metal implants or bone grafts in a procedure called spinal fusion. Although fusion helps to strengthen and stabilize the cervical spine, it limits movement of the neck. It also puts added stress on the vertebrae above and below the fusion. The artificial disc, made of stainless steel, replaces the impaired natural disc removed during discectomy. Compared with fusion surgery, an artificial disc should allow for greater movement of the spine and reduce stress and deterioration of adjacent vertebrae.

In one study of individuals with cervical degenerative disc disease who received either standard discectomy or artificial disc replacement, researchers found that while participants in both groups had less neck and arm pain five years after surgery, those in the artificial disc replacement group recovered faster and had significantly less neck pain and disability and better general health than those who had fusion surgery. X-rays revealed deterioration of adjacent vertebrae in about one in three patients in the artificial disc replacement group, compared with about half of patients who had fusion surgery. More fusion surgery patients required a second surgical procedure during the study period, primarily because of deterioration.

Disc transplants. Disc transplants are under study as well. One small, preliminary trial in China involved 13 individuals with cervical disc herniation whose damaged discs were surgically removed and replaced with discs from young adults who had died. After an average of six years, the transplant recipients had less pain and a 68% improvement in neurological function. And although there were signs of mild degeneration in the new discs, the motion and stability of the spine were preserved. The authors concluded that with further refinements, transplantation could be an effective treatment. Still, this technique must be tested on many more individuals before it becomes widely available.

Radiofrequency neurotomy. Radiofrequency neurotomy is another pain relief option for people whose neck pain can be confirmed (via a facet joint injection) to originate in a cervical facet joint. In this treatment, an electric current is applied to the nerve that serves the offending facet joint. The nerve is damaged so that it no longer conducts pain signals, but it is not permanently destroyed. The effects of radiofrequency neurotomy may last from nine to 18 months, at which point the procedure may be repeated. Radiofrequency neurotomy is a technically difficult procedure. It is usually reserved for people with chronic, significant pain that has not responded to other treatments.

Toward a pain-free future

Doctors are constantly striving to improve the diagnosis, treatment, and prevention of neck pain. Clinical trials are under way involving exercise, massage, and chiropractic medicine, in addition to high-tech surgical innovations and research using 3D printing to create a scaffold for growing replacement discs.

In the meantime, there is a lot you and your doctor can do to manage and relieve your pain today, beginning with exercise, physical therapy, and the simple lifestyle adjustments described in the Special Section of this report. Whether you ultimately need physical therapy, medication, or surgery, the options available right now can go a long way toward easing your discomfort—and relieving that proverbial pain in the neck. ■

Resources

Organizations

American Academy of Orthopaedic Surgeons
9400 W. Higgins Road
Rosemont, IL 60018
847-823-7186
www.aaos.org
www.orthoinfo.org (for patient information only)

This professional organization for orthopedic surgeons provides fact sheets and booklets on numerous neck and back problems. The website includes a physician locator.

American College of Rheumatology
2200 Lake Blvd. NE
Atlanta, GA 30319
404-633-3777
www.rheumatology.org

This professional organization for specialists in arthritis and related conditions provides fact sheets on back pain, fibromyalgia, and several types of arthritis. The website includes a physician locator.

American Massage Therapy Association
500 Davis St., Suite 900
Evanston, IL 60201
877-905-0577 (toll-free)
www.amtamassage.org

This professional association for massage therapists offers a therapist locator service on its website.

American Physical Therapy Association
1111 N. Fairfax St.
Alexandria, VA 22314
800-999-2782 (toll-free)
www.apta.org

This national professional organization for physical therapists provides information on preventing and treating neck pain and on maintaining good posture throughout life. The website includes a therapist locator service.

American Society for the Alexander Technique
11 W. Monument Ave., Suite 510
Dayton, OH 45402
800-473-0620 (toll-free)
www.amsatonline.org

This national professional organization for Alexander Technique teachers provides information on the lessons and how they are applied. The website includes a locator for certified teachers.

Arthritis Foundation
1355 Peachtree St. NE, 6th floor
Atlanta, GA 30309
800-283-7800 (toll-free)
www.arthritis.org

This nonprofit organization produces more than 100 consumer publications, and its website offers extensive information on arthritis and fibromyalgia.

Biofeedback Certification International Alliance
5310 Ward Road, Suite 201
Arvada, CO 80002
720-502-5829
www.bcia.org

This organization certifies practitioners in biofeedback. Its website offers general information on biofeedback and a search engine to find practitioners with various specialties, including physical therapy, neuromuscular rehabilitation, and pain.

National Certification Commission for Acupuncture and Oriental Medicine
76 S. Laura St., Suite 1290
Jacksonville, FL 32202
904-598-1005
www.nccaom.org

This organization provides certification of practitioners in acupuncture. Its website is designed for acupuncture professionals, but it does provide a search engine to find acupuncture practitioners by region.

North American Spine Society
7075 Veterans Blvd.
Burr Ridge, IL 60527
630-230-3600
www.spine.org

This is a multidisciplinary medical organization for spine care professionals. The website offers information about spine conditions and treatments as well as a spine care provider search.

Harvard Special Health Reports

The following Special Health Reports from Harvard Medical School elaborate on topics mentioned briefly in this report. To order, go to www.health.harvard.edu or call 877-649-9457 (toll-free).

Back Pain: Finding solutions for your aching back
Jeffrey N. Katz, M.D., Medical Editor
(Harvard Medical School, 2014)

Back pain has many causes and, as a result, many treatments. This report describes the different types of back problems and the tailored treatments that are more likely to help specific conditions, with particular emphasis on lower back pain.

Core Exercises: 5 workouts to tighten your abs, strengthen your back, and improve your balance
Lauren E. Elson, M.D., Medical Editor, with
Michele Stanten, Fitness Consultant
(Harvard Medical School, 2016)

Building your core is about more than strengthening your abs. It's about building up the muscles in the back, abdomen, pelvis, buttocks, and hips that undergird almost everything you do, from sitting up straight to playing sports. Core exercises help you strengthen your core muscles and, in the process, improve your posture and reduce neck strain.

Gentle Core Exercises: Start toning your abs, building your back muscles, and reclaiming core fitness today
Edward M. Phillips, M.D., Medical Editor, with Josie Gardiner, Personal Trainer
(Harvard Medical School, 2014)

This report presents a gentle program of core exercises that lets you get started in a safe, easy way, if you've had an injury, you've been unwell, or you're not ready to start with a tougher program, like the one in the *Core Exercises* Special Health Report.

Living Well with Osteoarthritis: A guide to keeping your joints healthy
Robert H. Shmerling, M.D., Medical Editor
(Harvard Medical School, 2016)

Osteoarthritis—the most common type of arthritis—is painful and can interfere with your ability to do things you enjoy. But there are many steps you can take to protect your joints, reduce discomfort, and improve mobility. This report covers the gamut, from established medical therapies to the use of assistive devices and complementary treatments such as acupuncture.

Rheumatoid Arthritis: How to protect your joints, reduce pain, and improve mobility
Robert H. Shmerling, M.D., Medical Editor
(Harvard Medical School, 2014)

Rheumatoid arthritis can cause unremitting joint pain, diminish joint function, and even rob you of your independence. This report explains the steps you can take to protect your joints, reduce discomfort, and improve your mobility. Because living with this disease involves more than finding a drug treatment, a special section provides advice about how to care for yourself through adaptations in your personal and work life.

Glossary

acupuncture: An ancient Chinese technique that uses slim needles to stimulate precise points along the body's "energy meridians" in order to relieve pain, among other purposes.

annulus: The tough outer covering of an intervertebral disc.

atlas: Another name for the C-1 vertebra of the neck, which lies just beneath the skull.

axis: Another name for the C-2 vertebra of the neck, which lies just beneath the C-1 vertebra.

brachial plexus: A network of nerves that are rooted at the cervical spine and provide sensation and movement to the shoulder and arm.

cervical radiculopathy: Compression of the spinal nerve roots in the neck, causing neurological symptoms such as tingling and numbness in the areas served by the nerves. Commonly known as a pinched nerve.

cervical spine: The portion of the spine located in the neck and consisting of the top seven vertebrae.

cervicogenic headache: Headache related to neck problems. Also called cervical headache.

degenerative disc disease: A general term for the age-related deterioration (loss of water and increased brittleness) of the cushioning discs between the vertebrae.

degenerative joint disease: See osteoarthritis.

disc: See intervertebral disc.

discectomy: The surgical removal of all or part of an intervertebral disc.

dislocation: An injury in which one of the bones of a joint is forced out of place.

facet joints: The paired joints located on the back side of each vertebra, connecting its back parts to those of the vertebrae above and below.

fibromyalgia: A syndrome characterized by musculoskeletal pain, poor sleep, fatigue, and tender joints.

herniated disc: A displacement of some portion of the intervertebral disc from its normal location; sometimes indicates a ruptured or "slipped" disc.

intervertebral disc: One of the small, energy-absorbing cushions between the vertebrae.

intervertebral foramen: The opening between vertebrae through which a spinal nerve exits the spinal column (plural: foramina).

lamina: One of the two thin, platelike parts of each vertebra that join in the midline and form the base of the spinous process of that vertebra (plural: laminae).

laminectomy: An operation in which all or part of one or both laminae is removed to gain access to the spinal canal or to decompress the spinal cord or nerve roots.

ligament: Fibrous tissue stabilizing and connecting bones to one another.

myelopathy: Disorder of the spinal cord.

osteoarthritis: A joint disease common with aging that is characterized by progressive deterioration of the cartilage lining the joints; also called degenerative joint disease.

osteophyte: An outgrowth of bone on the margins of a joint or intervertebral disc, known informally as a bone spur; generally a result of osteoarthritis.

pinched nerve: See cervical radiculopathy.

posterior keyhole foraminotomy: A minimally invasive surgical procedure that is sometimes an option for repairing a herniated disc.

spinal fusion: A procedure to join two or more vertebrae with a bone graft in order to eliminate motion and relieve pain.

spinal stenosis: A narrowing of the canal in which the spinal cord lies.

spondylosis: A general term for degeneration of the spine.

sprain: Injury to a ligament that may involve overstretching and the development of small tears.

strain: Injury to a muscle, with overstretching or the development of small tears, caused by misuse or overuse.

tendinitis: Inflammation of the tendons.

transcutaneous electrical nerve stimulation (TENS): Use of low-voltage electrical current to provide pain-suppressing stimulation.

trigger point: A painful area that, when stimulated, also elicits pain elsewhere in the body—such as the arm, the shoulder, or another area of the neck.

vertebra: One of the cylindrical bones that form the spine (plural: vertebrae).

vertebral foramen: The hole in the center of each vertebra (plural: foramina).

whiplash: The popular term for muscle and ligament damage resulting from rapid and extreme extension and flexion of the neck. The term is also used for the accident causing the injury—most often a rear-end motor vehicle accident.